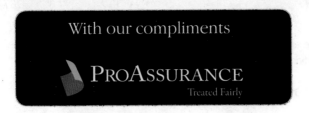
—— Third Edition ——

ICD-10 DOCUMENTATION STRATEGIES TO SUPPORT SEVERITY OF ILLNESS

Ensure an Accurate Professional Profile

Robert S. Gold, MD

D0912633

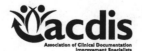
acdis
Association of Clinical Documentation
Improvement Specialists

ICD-10 Documentation Strategies to Support Severity of Illness: Ensure an Accurate Professional Profile, Third Edition, is published by HCPro, a division of BLR.

Robert S. Gold, MD, Author
Gloryanne Bryant, RHIA, CDIP, CCS,
    CCDS, Reviewer
Gerianne Spanek, Managing Editor
Erin Callahan, Senior Director, Product

Melissa Osborn, Product Director
Mike Mirabello, Production Specialist
Matt Sharpe, Senior Manager of Production
Shane Katz, Art Director
Elizabeth Petersen, Vice President

HCPro, a division of BLR
75 Sylvan Street, Suite A-101
Danvers, MA 01923
Telephone: 800-650-6787 or 781-639-1872
Fax: 800-639-8511
Email: *customerservice@hcpro.com*

Visit HCPro online at *www.hcpro.com* and *www.hcmarketplace.com*.

11/2013
22061

Contents

About the Author

Robert S. Gold, MD

Robert S. Gold has more than 40 years of experience as a physician, medical director, and consultant. A graduate of Hahnemann Medical College in Philadelphia, he trained in general surgery in the U.S. Navy, where he spent his professional career as a practicing surgeon.

Since leaving military service, Dr. Gold has worked as a consultant in the fields of managed care medicine, locum tenens, home healthcare, and hospital accreditation and licensure. Most notably, during the past 16 years, his work has focused on educational programs pertaining to documentation, coding, and billing accuracy for healthcare services.

Dr. Gold is known nationally for his educational presentations regarding the clinical orientation of coding in American Health Information Management Association and HCPro audio conferences. He has spoken about medical staff participation in clinical documentation improvement (CDI) programs at national and state-level health information management association and Association of Clinical Documentation Improvement Specialists meetings. He writes the monthly columns *Clinically Speaking* for Briefings on Coding Compliance Strategies and *Minute for the Medical Staff* for Medical Records Briefing, both published by HCPro, a division of BLR.

Dr. Gold is a cofounder of DCBA, Inc., an Atlanta consulting firm that provides physician-led CDI programs, educating integrated teams of medical staff members, CDI specialists, and coders. His programs lead to increased compliance, proper reflection of true severity of illness, and improved morbidity and mortality statistics for the hospitals and their medical staff.

Contact him at *RGold@DCBAInc.com.*

About the Reviewer

Gloryanne Bryant, RHIA, CDIP, CCS, CCDS

Gloryanne Bryant is a sought-after national speaker and author on healthcare compliance, reimbursement, clinical documentation improvement (CDI), and coding regulations. With more than 30 years of experience in health information management (HIM), she serves as a catalyst for change and improvement in HIM and healthcare.

A past president of the California Health Information Association (CHIA), Bryant has conducted numerous workshops for hospital-based coders, addressing ICD-9-CM, ICD-10-CM/PCS, and CPT® coding; diagnosis-related groups (DRG); and ambulatory payment classification (APC) outpatient prospective payment system (OPPS). She is an American Health Information Management Association (AHIMA)–approved ICD-10-CM/PCS trainer.

Bryant has made numerous presentations on data quality, medical necessity, compliance, and CDI to management executives and healthcare administrators. She was the keynote speaker at the 2013 AHIMA CDI Summit and has been a guest speaker on compliance issues for regional, state, and national educational programs and associations. She has given presentations on ICD-10 planning and implementation and provided testimony in support of ICD-10 implementation to the U.S. House Ways and Means Committee in April 2006.

Bryant serves as a volunteer leader on many levels. She has served as a director and president-elect of CHIA and has served in several national positions for AHIMA. She also served on the American Hospital Association editorial advisory board on ICD-9-CM for *Coding Clinic* for two years.

Bryant received the CHIA Literary Award for her many articles and other writing related to CDI, compliance, data quality, and coding. She worked on OPPS policy, coding, and reimbursement issues as a member of the Centers for Medicare & Medicaid Services APC Advisory Panel from August 2005 until August 2009. She also served on the RAND Expert Panel on Severity DRGs from 2006 to 2007. She received the AHIMA Triumph Award in the category of HIM Champion in 2007.

Bryant is the national director of coding quality, education, systems, and support for national revenue cycle of Kaiser Permanente and national revenue cycle co-lead of ICD-10 coding education and training. Based in Oakland, Calif., Bryant is also an advisor to CDI programs and staff.

ICD-10 Documentation Strategies to Support Severity of Illness: Ensure an Accurate Professional Profile, Third Edition

Introduction

Physicians in the United States are becoming more aware of the value of clinical data and the relationships between their professional profiles and the International Classification of Diseases (ICD) and Current Procedural Terminology (CPT®) codes they assign, or those assigned for them by others. Certainly, internists are aware of the value of personal professional billing codes, and surgeons are aware of their morbidity and mortality rates. These all relate to the ICD codes assigned for diagnoses, treatments, and procedures performed.

If the clinical documentation and, thus, the codes do not accurately and specifically represent the work a physician does, someone can be inconvenienced—if not actually hurt—with data that poorly reflects on the practitioner's quality of care.

The healthcare industry has entered a new era of value based purchasing (VBP), in which a healthcare provider's statistics will determine whether the provider is preferred or to be avoided. Medicare started the initiative a few years ago, and in 2012, it took its first giant steps. Private insurance companies have jumped aboard and are making their determinations of selection of physicians and hospitals to be utilized by their clients based on data. The elements of this data include:

- Cooperation with official practice guidelines for acute myocardial infarction (AMI), heart failure (HF), pneumonia (PNA), postoperative wound infections, and avoidance of deep vein thrombosis (DVT) after surgeries

- Severity-adjusted mortality rates

- Severity-adjusted complication rates (patient safety)

  - Frequency of patient safety indicators occurring

  - Frequency of "never" events

  - Frequency of postoperative and postprocedural complications

- Severity-adjusted length of stay and patient costs

  - Appropriate venue for delivery of healthcare

  - Avoidance of preventable readmissions to hospital

- Bundled payments

  - Combined payments between hospital and physician for inpatient care

  - Combined payments for outpatient element of patients after hospitalization

- Combined payments for global care of patients

- Combined, severity-adjusted payments between surgeons and facility

All of these measures are determined through analysis of ICD codes, and an understanding of how the physician's documentation justifies assignment of the correct ICD codes is paramount for future success of a practice.

Finally, on October 1, 2014, the United States joins the other nations that already use the International Classification of Diseases system, 10th revision (ICD-10), which requires even greater attention to documentation and assignment of ICD codes than ever before. Physician survival in this new value-based world will depend on documentation and assignment of accurate and specific ICD-10 codes. Both will be paramount to success.

Professional organizations have begun working to help their physician members understand how clinical documentation and ICD codes derived from that documentation affect quality of care. Physicians must understand that these codes explain the mental work they do to determine their patients' current health problems and ongoing health status. The complexity of a physician's medical decision-making reflects the complexity of the patient, and the terms that physicians use in the medical record—whether in the hospital, the office, or in a skilled nursing facility—lead to code assignments that either do or do not inform the database that they know their patients.

All physicians took courses in pathology and physiology and learned about causes of symptoms and specific etiologies of disease manifestations. However, physicians often take shortcuts with respect to the clinical documentation in their patients' medical records, and those shortcuts hurt not only their profiles but the United States and its overall healthcare system.

The Uniform Hospital Discharge Data Set (UHDDS) requires hospitals to report conditions that affect patient care and require clinical evaluation, therapeutic treatment, diagnostic procedures, extended length of hospital stay, and increased nursing care/monitoring. Identifying these components of the conditions adds to the complexity of medical decision-making and enhances severity profiles.

Physicians and the hospital health information management (HIM) department must communicate and collaborate with each other. The HIM coding staff must have an opportunity to ask physicians questions or to request clarification when clinical documentation is not specific. A strong partnership between physicians, HIM staff, and clinical documentation improvement staff is also an imperative for success.

Due to increased regulatory scrutiny of clinical documentation to support medical necessity and coding, documentation that is complete, specific, and detailed will serve as a good defense.

This book will help physicians understand many of the specific diagnosis-related issues—and relieve them of much of the rework associated with utilization review, case management, HIM/medical records issues, and questions from those who oversee their work.

This book is not all-inclusive. Instead, it serves as a guide to improving clinical documentation and to capturing acuity, severity of illness (SOI), and risk of mortality (ROM) for the patients that physicians serve.

Acute Myocardial Infarction

Classification of acute myocardial infarction (MI) has two major categories:

- **Type 1**—Acute myocardial infarction caused by acute occlusion of a coronary artery by thrombus, embolism, or ruptured athero-sclerotic plaque

- **Type 2**—Demand acute myocardial infarction whereby no acute occlusive process has taken place but demand for oxygenated blood to avoid death of some myocardial cells exceeds the body's capabilities of supplying that resource

MIs are also classified as follows:

- **Type 3**—Associated with sudden cardiac death, such that the physician does not know whether an MI caused a fatal arrhythmia or an arrhythmia caused the MI.

- **Type 4**—MIs that occur related to a current angioplasty with or without stent. Depending on the clinical circumstances, it may not require intervention if it is small, or it may be significant and require further intervention.

- 4a occurs early after placement of a stent and is often associated with malposition or movement of the stent or subintimal dissection

- 4b occurs later but is still related to the angioplasty and placement of the stent

- **Type 5**—MIs that occur related to a current coronary artery bypass procedure.

In Types 4 and 5, if not clinically significant, no complication documentation or code should be considered. If increased treatment or other intervention for an adverse patient outcome from the post-procedural MI is required, documentation relating to a cardiac complication of surgery should be provided. Consequently, a code should be assigned to track it.

Result

- ST-elevation MI (**STEMI**), which usually occurs with Type 1 mechanism but can also occur with Type 2, 4 or 5 events. For those patients who are not excluded, STEMI requires that they be entered into the nationally accepted practice guidelines for acute STEMI. Patients with a demand ST-elevation MI generally have a near occlusive lesion of a coronary artery to begin with but no acute occlusion. They should also be included in the practice guidelines.

- Non-ST-elevation MI (**NSTEMI**), which can occur because of a Type 1 or Type 2 mechanism.

Clinical criteria for identifying acute demand myocardial infarction

- Symptoms of acute MI (either typical presentation with chest pain or atypical without chest pain).

- Clinical circumstances consistent with acute demand (e.g., shock, severe acute anemia, hypoxia, tachyarrhythmia, accelerated hypertension).

- A significant spike in troponin level with at least one reading higher than top normal for the laboratory. (Three equally elevated troponins do not signify an acute MI. This usually identifies a chronic condition [e.g., significant sustained bradycardia, end-stage renal disease, hypertrophic cardiomyopathy].)

Documentation needs

- After workup, did the patient likely have an MI (NSTEMI or STEMI)? (Documentation is inadequate if you state "acute coronary syndrome with troponinemia" or "demand ischemia.") Fulfilling the documentation needs for the "acute" episode of MI will help improve outcomes.

- If STEMI, was there cardiogenic shock present and documented? Or is there a new left bundle branch block? (Check whether vital signs show significantly low blood pressure and whether a ventricular assist device or pressors were used.) Was the new left bundle branch block documented in the medical record, and not just on the EKG (electrocardiogram)?

- If demand MI, what was the causative factor (e.g., atrial fibrillation [AF] with rapid ventricular response [RVR] or other tachyarrhythmia, severe chronic anemia or acute anemia and the cause of the anemia, or hypoxia or hypoperfusion, and from what source)?

- Did the patient present with congestive heart failure (CHF)? If acute, seek clarification. (Check whether the brain natriuretic peptide [BNP] is elevated, whether there is presence of rales or shortness of breath, or whether an x-ray shows pulmonary edema, because this may indicate that a physician query is necessary.) Was it acute systolic heart failure with new drop in EF (ejection fraction) to less than 40%, or was it acute diastolic heart failure (normal ejection fraction)?

- Did the patient develop pericarditis or other post-MI symptoms, such as post-MI fever or post-MI leukocytosis (signs of Dressler's syndrome), or was there post-MI angina? (Document whether there is continued chest pain after the MI and its cause.)

- Did the patient have an arrhythmia during the hospital stay that was not documented and that may or may not have required treatment? If so, identify that arrhythmia and the decision-making.

- When documentation is not clear as to the acuity of the MI, answer these questions:

  - Is this the first hospitalization for this acute MI?

  - Did the patient have the MI before admission, or did it occur after admission? Document the principal diagnoses that led to the decision to admit.

- Was there a second MI during this or a recent hospitalization, and did it occur within four weeks of a previous one?

Background heart disease

- Does the patient have background heart disease with right heart failure (chronic cor pulmonale) or chronic left ventricular systolic or diastolic heart failure (check echo for EF with dilation of left ventricle [systolic dysfunction with EF + 40%] or modeling of hypertrophy [normal EF with or without diastolic dysfunction respectively])?

- Is it documented as due to ischemic cardiomyopathy, valvular disease (valvular cardiomyopathy), hypertensive heart disease (or hypertensive cardiomyopathy), alcoholic cardiomyopathy, amyloid heart, viral cardiomyopathy, toxic cardiomyopathy (and from what drug), hypertrophic cardiomyopathy, or unknown cause?

- Document your impression or answer(s) to the question(s) in progress notes and upon discharge.

Refer to the Heart Failure section for additional information.

Adverse Effects of Medications

Background and clinical implications

Medications sometimes have side effects that can lead to discomfort or functional abnormalities that will mimic other diseases, such as nausea and vomiting, diarrhea, or drop in blood pressure with syncope or acute renal failure. Sometimes, drugs have cumulative effects—that is, one does not cause a significant abnormality, but along with other drugs, it can create symptoms, such as alteration of consciousness or shortness of breath, that seem to indicate another disease. Sometimes a patient experiences a life-threatening event that rarely occurs in the general population.

Finally, sometimes while achieving the desired effect, the drug causes another condition that a patient has to become significantly worse, such as gastrointestinal bleeding, hematuria in a patient on warfarin, or acute respiratory failure from worsening chronic obstructive pulmonary disease (COPD) in a hypertensive patient on beta-blockers.

- An adverse effect is a clinical problem that occurs when a drug is given to the proper patient in the proper dosage and is taken properly by the patient. A poisoning occurs (for the purpose of capturing coded data) when the wrong patient takes the medication or the right patient takes an overdose.

- When a medical workup demonstrates that a patient's presenting symptoms on admission are due to side effects or adverse effects of a medicine taken properly, the presenting condition is sequenced as the hospital principal diagnosis, and an E-code (adverse effect code) is assigned later to show which drug or class of drug led to the effect.

Note: **Warfarin** (Coumadin™) **toxicity** is not poisoning unless a patient takes the wrong dosage. The effect (high prothrombin time or international normalized ratio [INR] level) or whatever is bleeding should be documented as the diagnosis, and code Z79.01 should be reported for long-term use of anticoagulants.

Phenytoin (Dilantin™) **toxicity** is not poisoning unless a patient takes the wrong dosage. The symptoms the patient presented with will be the principal diagnosis (e.g., nausea and vomiting, alteration of consciousness) in this situation.

The most important detail is the **documented link of the presenting symptoms** or **the worsening of the presentation to the specific drug(s)**.

Documentation needs

- Document the patient's signs and symptoms of the adverse effect of the medication you believe to be the cause with the term *due to*.

- Document drug–drug interactions; specifically, identify the drugs and the adverse effect.

- Document patients who take multiple drugs and who may experience multiple side effects. Specify whether this is the cause of specific symptoms.

- Document predisposing factors, such as other diseases, dietary issues, or over-the-counter drug use.

- When respiratory depression is due to drug use, specify/document whether the case involved the proper dose, an overdose, or use of illicit or illegal drugs. (The latter are poisonings rather than adverse effects because there is usually no prescribed dosage by a physician.)

Alcohol and Substance Use and Abuse

Background

Patients may present to the hospital with symptoms related to current use of alcohol or illicit drugs or with other conditions that can be tied to the patient's recent acute or habitual use of these substances. The specificity of the pattern of use and the link of the symptoms to the substance use is fundamental.

- **Abuse** implies overuse of alcohol or any use of illicit drugs without implication of dependence. Abuse can be *episodic* (e.g., weekends only) or *continuous* (e.g., daily). These are classified by the specific drug or drug group used by the patient (e.g., marijuana, hallucinogens, opiates, cocaine).

- **Dependence** is similarly classified to overuse of alcohol or of a specific illicit substance. This term implies that use is more than recreational and that the patient's lifestyle is affected by the presence or absence of the dependent substance. This is similarly specified in the coding classification as *continuous* or *episodic* use.

Documentation needs

- Clarify/document in the medical record when a patient sometimes consumes alcohol but does not have an abuse or dependence problem (e.g., cite social drinking or volume of wine, beer, or other and frequency).

- Specify/document whether the patient has a history of alcohol problems (e.g., heavy drinking in the past but not at present), whether the case involves periodic or episodic abuse (e.g., weekend drinker), or whether the patient is alcohol-dependent.

- Specify/document whether other body systems are affected by alcohol or drug abuse or dependence and identify the related disease process (e.g., sleep disorders, psychosis, sexual dysfunction, amnestic disorders, dementia).

- Document whether you think a patient is an occasional abuser or is dependent on alcohol or illegal or controlled drugs.

- Document whether the patient suffers from substance abuse and identify the substance. Writing (+) coc or (+) barb or (-) ETOH has no clinical significance. In accordance with coding guidelines, coding staff may not assign codes based on a positive laboratory test.

- Identify whether a link exists between the identified drug abuse or dependence and organ malfunction, such as alcoholic cardiomyopathy, alcoholic cirrhosis, or chest pain due to cocaine abuse.

- Clarify manifestations on withdrawal, such as delirium, hallucinations, and perceptual disturbances.

Anemia

Clinical criteria

Clinical criteria include a hemoglobin level that is below low normal for your laboratory (most physicians use 10 as a general rule). A drop in hemoglobin level without achieving anemia does not require questioning, but it may require defining and documenting the cause of the drop in hemoglobin.

Mechanisms

- **Congenital disease**—Sickle cell, thalassemia, spherocytosis, ellipticytosis, glucose-6-phosphatase dehydrogenase deficiency.

- **Nutrient deficiency**—Iron deficiency (microcytic, hypochromic red cells), vitamin B_{12} (macrocytic anemia), severe protein malnutrition.

- **Chronic blood loss**—Gastrointestinal (GI) blood loss, chronic hematuria, chronic menometrorrhagia.

- **Acute blood loss**—Due to a disease, such as acute GI bleed, rupture of aneurysm or other vessel tear, spleen or liver rupture, severe scalp laceration, fracture of femur, or associated with an operation involving large volumes of blood loss, such as aortic aneurysm surgery or liver surgery.

- **Complication of a surgical procedure**—Operation usually associated with small volumes of blood loss may entail massive blood loss due to inadvertent events (e.g., tear of a major vein, avulsion of spleen, unplanned entry into the aorta or major artery), which may result in anemia from acute blood loss.

- **Chronic kidney disease (CKD)**—Usually stage 3 or higher with glomerular filtration rate (GFR) under 45 ml/min.

- **Specific other chronic disease** such as hepatitis or chronic osteomyelitis (identify condition).

- **Chemotherapy**—Check whether platelets and white count are also low in cases of transient pancytopenia or long-term aplastic anemia; name chemotherapy drug.

- **Bone marrow malignancy**—Neoplasm in the bone marrow or of the bone marrow.

- **Myelodysplastic condition.**

- **Hemodilution only** may lead to drop in hemoglobin, especially in patients after dialysis or surgery on patients with autonomic nerve dysfunction, and does not represent anemia at all. It is often not treated.

Thought processes

- Patients may have multiple factors in play at any time, and you must specify/document them.

- A significant drop in hemoglobin may indicate acute blood loss, but the patient may not develop anemia.

- A drop in hemoglobin may be due to hemodilution from large volumes of crystalloid and not represent anemia at all.

- Hemoglobin level could start within the normal range for the patient's gender and drop to below normal (below 10). If there is an indication bleeding has occurred, it is reasonable to determine that the patient has anemia due to acute blood loss.

- Hemoglobin level could start below normal and drop significantly lower, in which case it may be anemia due to some chronic cause, in addition to anemia due to acute blood loss.

Acute GI bleed, acute menorrhagia, acute onset of gross hematuria, and **acute retroperitoneal hematoma** all imply "acute blood loss." Therefore, no additional clarification is necessary to determine that there was blood loss, but you must include in your documentation the "acute" level.

A low hemoglobin level with no significant change implies a chronic anemic condition. Only cases associated with known chronic bleeding may be considered to represent anemia due to chronic blood loss.

Note of gastroenterologic importance: Newly found iron deficiency anemia in an elderly patient is cancer of the right colon until proven otherwise.

Documentation needs

- Document whether the patient has anemia due to blood loss from a disease process, and identify the disease process and the acuity or chronicity of the bleed (e.g., anemia due to acute blood loss from fractured femur, anemia due to chronic blood loss from right colon cancer).

- Document whether the patient is anemic due to another cause (e.g., end-stage renal disease [ESRD]) or bone marrow suppression) and document an explanation of the link (e.g., anemia of ESRD, anemia from chemotherapy, anemia due to chronic osteomyelitis).

- In addition to anemia, clarify in your documentation whether a patient has transient pancytopenia due to chemotherapeutic agents or other specific drug, or whether it has resulted in long-term or permanent aplastic anemia.

- Document whether a patient develops anemia from excessive blood loss from the GI tract or the urinary tract, due to retroperitoneal bleed or being on long-term coagulants, or during surgery due to a true hematologic problem.

- Clarify whether a bleeding episode was prolonged because patient was receiving anticoagulant therapy, and identify the medication.

- Document the factors of which you are aware that have contributed to the patient's case of multifactorial anemia and identify each one.

- Document whether a patient has excessive blood loss during a procedure due to a complication, such as inadvertent entry into the femoral vein during a herniorrhaphy.

Atrial Arrhythmias: Fibrillation, Flutter

Background

These are common arrhythmias that, alone, do not often cause symptoms or difficulties in performing normal daily activities. However, they can lead to severe complications such as bradycardia with syncope, tachycardia with unstable angina or non ST-elevation demand myocardial infraction or acute pulmonary edema, embolism with resultant stroke, acute intestinal ischemia, or embolism to the legs.

They may be associated with or caused by cardiac ischemic events in the past, trauma to the heart, inflammation of the heart, thyroid disorders (hypothyroidism or hyperthyroidism), mitral valve disease, or alcoholism. Their presence is best identified by character of occurrence in fibrillation and in typicality of rhythm and sites of origin in cases of flutter. The two conditions may coexist in the same patient. Either may be treated medically or with electrophysiologic study and ablation of sources of the abnormal beat pattern or with valvular surgery if necessary.

Typical atrial flutter generally indicates a single focus of irritability with stable abnormal heart rate. Atypical flutter indicates varying foci of irritability with varying abnormal heart rates. The route that the electrical impulses take is typical or atypical, and that will be shown in EP (electrophysiologic) studies.

Documentation needs

- Identify significant arrhythmias on EKG not identified in progress notes.

- Identify cause of atrial fibrillation or atrial flutter, if known.

- Clarify whether tachycardia or bradycardia associated with the arrhythmia caused the patient's presentation (e.g., unstable angina, NSTEMI, acute diastolic heart failure, acute pulmonary edema, sudden cardiac death).

- Clarify whether embolic phenomenon (e.g., stroke, intestinal, leg) originated from left atrial appendage clot seen on echocardiogram.

- Clarify whether tachy-brady syndrome exists based on serial EKGs demonstrating widely variant ventricular rates in case of atrial fibrillation.

- In cases of atrial fibrillation, clarify whether paroxysmal, persistent, or chronic.

- In cases of atrial flutter, clarify whether typical or atypical flutter exists.

- Does the patient have both atrial fibrillation and atrial flutter? If so, clarify/document each separately, if known.

Chest Pain and Angina

Chest pain can have numerous causes. The most important thing for a physician to determine is whether the chest pain represents an acute myocardial infarction (MI). Once that is ruled out (usually by electrocardiogram or lack of rise in troponin level), other cardiac or noncardiac causes of chest pain must be determined. Often, the specific cause is never identified.

Cardiac causes

- Acute MI (see Acute Myocardial Infarction)

- **Unstable angina** due to _____ (the link is of paramount importance)

- Coronary atherosclerotic disease (CAD)

- Aortic stenosis

- Hypertrophic cardiomyopathy

- Pulmonary artery hypertension

- Severe anemia (acute or progressive chronic pain relieved with transfusion)

- Tachyarrhythmia (AF with RVR, supraventricular tachycardia, pain relieved with slowing heart rate)

- Hypertensive emergency (accelerated or malignant hypertension, pain relieved with dropping blood pressure)

- Thyroid storm

- Any shock or significant hypovolemia

- Stable angina

- Pericarditis (with or without effusion)

- Myocarditis

Noncardiac causes

- Pulmonary embolism (from deep vein thrombosis, fat embolism, air embolism)

- Costochondritis (reproducible pain with pressure on costal cartilage)

- Gastroesophageal reflux

- Rib fracture or other chest trauma

- Pneumonia/pleurisy

- Lung cancer

- Acute cholecystitis or hepatitis

Documentation needs

- Document the origin of the chest pain (i.e., cardiac, noncardiac). If angina, specify/document whether stable, unstable, acute MI, acute pericarditis, myocardial contusion.

- Document the primary source of the angina, if known (e.g., CAD, aortic stenosis, hypertrophic cardiomyopathy, pulmonary artery hypertension, Prinzmetal coronary spasm).

- Document whether the pain represents secondary cause of unstable angina and specify whether due to tachyarrhythmia, bradycardia, anemia, or metabolic demands, such as thyrotoxicosis.

- Specify/document whether chest pain is related to a condition such as musculoskeletal disease, pleuritic disease, gastroesophageal reflux disease (GERD), gallbladder disease, or Tietze syndrome, if known.

Chronic Obstructive Pulmonary Disease

Background

Chronic obstructive pulmonary disease (COPD) can be a chronic, stable condition or can present with acute symptoms of shortness of breath, cough, and, frequently, wheezing (called exacerbation of COPD).

Causes

- Inhalation of smoke or chemicals (e.g., cigarettes, anthracosis, other irritants).

- Repeated aspiration of gastric content, caused by chronic aspiration bronchitis.

- Prolonged, repeated severe asthma attacks.

- Emphysema.

- Bronchiectasis.

- Severity of chronic COPD ranges from mild to severe. If a patient has severe COPD or end-stage COPD, presence of chronic respiratory failure must be considered.

- Severity of acute exacerbation ranges from outpatient treatment to treatments in the emergency department to acute respiratory failure, which may require ventilatory support.

Clinical criteria

- Acute respiratory failure
  - Documented evidence of difficulty in breathing: use of accessory muscles of respiration, inability to speak more than two-word sentences, tachypnea (over 24 breaths/minute), cyanosis

  - Hypoxemic (Type 1) respiratory failure: SaO_2 cannot be maintained at 90% with 6 L of oxygen or $pO_2 < 60$ on room air

- Hypercapnic (Type 2) respiratory failure: pH < 7.30, pCO_2 > 50

- Chronic respiratory failure

  - pH normal with pCO_2 > 50

  - Polycythemia

  - Chronic cor pulmonale

  - Clubbing of fingers

  - Hypoxemic (Type 1) respiratory failure: pO_2 < 60 on room air

  - Hypercapnic (Type 2) respiratory failure: pH 7.40, pCO_2 > 50

Documentation needs

- Document whether the patient has acute bronchitis, acute exacerbation of chronic bronchitis, stable COPD, or other chronic lung disease.

- Document whether the patient has acute exacerbation of chronic asthmatic bronchitis when chronic asthma has led to chronic lung disease.

- Document whether the patient had acute respiratory failure upon admission, even if intubation was not necessary.

- Document whether the patient has chronic respiratory failure and needs home oxygen and other treatments while also meeting the above criteria.

- Document the likely etiology of this acute event (e.g., allergy, cold, viral or bacterial bronchitis, pneumonia).

- Document whether the patient's exacerbation was likely caused by aspiration (e.g., gross or microaspiration related to GERD or laryngeal dysfunction) and requires evaluation or treatment of the aspiration risk (e.g., aspiration bronchitis or aspiration pneumonitis). Differentiate from chronic restrictive lung disease as may occur with kyphoscoliosis, pectus excavatum, and morbid obesity with or without obesity hypoventilation syndrome.

Comfort Measures Only

Rationale

Patient and family desires regarding the extent of intervention for a terminal or dying patient while in the hospital has many levels. Assignment of **do not resuscitate (DNR)** status may vary from providing all care needed for all conditions that the patient develops short of intubation and mechanical ventilation to refusal of any medical interaction whatsoever. The assignment of **comfort measures only** ICD-10 code Z51.5 is a status usually arrived at with coordination of the stated desires of the patient, family, and physician, often with pastoral support.

Palliative services may be provided by a hospital team for any patient who requires ongoing treatment after discharge. The mere involvement of the palliative care team or palliative care consultation does not qualify for comfort measures only. Palliative care or comfort measures only provided to prepare the patient for imminent death do qualify.

Comfort measures may include hydration, pain control, drugs to control seizure activity, or any intervention to prevent the dying patient from becoming agitated and more uncomfortable. Antibiotics and any other drug used to treat a condition other than to keep the patient comfortable will be discontinued. Often, the situation involves removing the patient from a ventilator and allowing death to ensue.

Documentation needs

- Document medical staff communication with the family (whether by the consulting physician, chaplain, or palliative care) with respect to "withdrawal of life support" or "keep the patient comfortable" or "agreed to let the patient die with dignity." Additionally, there should be clear intent of documentation regarding DNR (or other similar terminology) within the medical record. Clarify whether this documentation meets your definition of comfort measures only or indicates intervention to be provided to the patient in case of change in status.

- If you request a palliative care consult (or inpatient hospice consult), document discussion with the patient or family and others regarding discontinuation of care. If you intend to maintain patient comfort with no further intervention, clarify whether the intent is comfort measures only or some limitation of response to change as in a DNR or other status.

Comorbidities or Comorbid Conditions

Rationale

Severity-adjusted data about physicians and hospitals are being collected. Severity-adjusted mortality risk or complication risk for surgeries will affect the surgical specialties more than ever before. When the physician managing a patient's care can document all of the patient's diseases on admission to the hospital and all coexisting acute or chronic conditions being treated, the severity of illness, risk of mortality, and complexity of medical decision-making are properly reflected.

For medical specialties, the comorbidities (patient's present diseases that are being managed, even though stable) affect the level of facility or professional billing for all admissions.

For surgical specialties, the comorbidities (other diseases that could potentially affect wound healing, recovery from anesthesia, and resistance to infection) are important data for the National Surgical Quality Improvement Project and the Society for Thoracic Surgery database.

Physicians should identify all diseases for which they order medications, even home medications, because they are responsible for the treatment of those diseases while the patient is in the hospital, regardless of the service for which the patient is admitted.

Documentation needs

- Document in the history and physical (H&P) whether the patient has other diseases that you or another physician are following, and identify the diseases.

- Document in the H&P the medications that the patient is currently taking and the diseases for which they are prescribed.

- Document all existing conditions (risk factors) that could affect the patient's ability to tolerate surgery, result in problems during or after surgery, or affect the hospitalization.

- Document in the discharge summary all conditions identified or clarified by consultants during your patient's hospital course.

- Identify/document a diagnosis whenever a patient's condition changes while the patient is in the hospital and you order tests or treatments.

- Document in the operative note any complications during the operation that require corrective action.

Complications: Postoperative

Background

Clinical conditions may be noted in the time period after an intervention, whether major surgical or procedural, that may not have been identified prior to the procedure. Sometimes, it is a matter of obtaining a more complete history of present illnesses after a surgical procedure has been performed. Sometimes, it will be a manifestation of the disease for which the surgery was performed. Other times, it will be an event that occurred in the operating suite due to the anesthesia or surgery.

Complications of surgery are conditions that follow an intervention and were caused by that intervention. Therefore, determining whether the diagnostic term reported in the postoperative period actually represented one of the previously described circumstances rather than having been a complication of the surgery is important. The coding data captures complications through the ICD-10-CM codes, which come from the clinical documentation.

Surgeons are measured by their complication statistics (i.e., morbidity and mortality rates). If they cause harm, capturing the cause and the effect is important. People often learn from mistakes or adverse events as a method of improving outcomes.

Anemia that may be found after surgery for a fracture of the neck of the femur is often due to the fracture, not the surgery. It could be referred to as **anemia due to acute blood loss from the femur fracture.** Similarly, anemia following surgery for a gastrointestinal bleed may be referred to as **anemia due to acute blood loss from the bleeding diverticulum.** Anemia after surgery caused by unplanned hemorrhage caused by the surgery is a complication of the surgical procedure and **the documentation must specifically state that a complication occurred.**

After **perforation of intestine** (e.g., diverticulum, appendix, gallbladder), ileus will occur because of the perforation and will prolong the postoperative recovery, but it represents ileus due to the perforated bowel and it should be documented as such. Adynamic or paralytic ileus is a normal consequence of an abdominal surgery and usually resolves in three to four days. **Ileus that prolongs the stay considerably beyond that or which results in reinsertion of a nasogastric tube may, indeed, be a complication of the surgery.** However, the coding staff must confirm that the patient did not have intestinal motility issues prior to the operative procedure, such as diabetic gastroparesis, which may have been the true cause of the prolonged ileus after the surgical procedure.

Documented events such as **wound infection, wound breakdown, excessive hemorrhage** from the wound and **hematomas** of significant size that require active treatment or significantly prolonged observation, **seromas, abscesses** after clean-clean surgery, and **pneumonia** (not present on admission or developing on admission) are always surgical complications. However, be sure to clarify when a surgical wound has purposely been left open, either to close secondarily or for return to the operating room at a later date for delayed primary closure. These are not wound infections or dehiscences.

If a surgeon or an internist who is following the case uses the documented term *postoperative* preceding a diagnosis (e.g., postoperative urinary retention, postoperative atelectasis), code assignment may result in a complication code. However, official coding guidelines state that a complication code should not be assigned just because of the presence of the word *postoperative*. Analysis to ensure the following before assignment of a complication code is important for coders and surgeons:

- The diagnostic condition was not caused by patient disease or medications

- The diagnostic condition met Uniform Hospital Discharge Data Set (UHDDS) criteria as a valid secondary diagnosis (clinically insignificant events should not be assigned complication codes)

- The diagnostic condition was not a complication of the anesthesia

- The diagnostic condition was not present on admission

- The diagnostic condition did not precede the procedure

- The diagnostic condition was not a normal part of events that occur after a procedure, and virtually all patients who undergo this procedure do not acquire this condition

If documentation of postoperative something appears in the progress notes, clarifying whether this was a complication of the procedure or providing some etiology to explain its presence (e.g., caused by the disease, caused by anesthesia, was present on admission but not identified at that time) is best practice.

Cor Pulmonale: Acute Due to Massive Pulmonary Embolism

Chronic cor pulmonale is usually manifested by right ventricular hypertrophy in response to chronic lung disease. In the face of a sudden and significant increase in pulmonary vascular resistance, such as massive pulmonary embolism or acute respiratory distress syndrome (ARDS), one may be faced with acute right heart failure associated with right ventricular dilation and acute respiratory failure.

Note that only 40% of patients with either of these conditions may develop acute cor pulmonale and require ventilatory and cardiotonic support.

Documentation needs

- Identify acute cor pulmonale when it exists.

- It is not synonymous with acute right heart failure or decompensated chronic cor pulmonale, and it is not caused by typical exacerbations of chronic obstrictive pulmonary disease (COPD) or pneumonia. Generally, an echocardiogram demonstrating dilation of the right ventricle validates this diagnosis.

- Identify the significant causative event.

- Ensure that you document the link.

Coronary Artery Disease

Identifying atherosclerosis of the coronary arteries as the cause of either a presenting symptom or of the disease process being treated is important. Specificity of the particular vessel involved, when known, is also crucial for data analysis. Coronary artery disease (CAD) is categorized as follows:

- Native vessel (always the correct designation when the patient has had no coronary artery surgery)

- Vein bypass

- Synthetic bypass

- Artery bypass (internal mammary)

- Native vessel of transplant heart

- Bypass vessel of transplant heart

- Unknown, native, or bypass vessel

Sometimes, long-term atherosclerotic disease of the coronaries can lead to long-term functional abnormality of the entire heart and result in heart failure (ischemic cardiomyopathy).

When a stent has been inserted in a coronary artery, designating whether obstruction at the stent is likely due to progression of the atherosclerosis in the stent or premature blockage occurred due to malpositioning of the stent (in-stent stenosis or end-stent stenosis) is important. Some stents will develop late obstruction due to the body's attempt to line the stent with cells usually found in the inner lining of native arteries; this is neointimal hyperplasia or overgrowth of the lining cells bridging the interior of the stent.

Documentation needs

- Specify/document whether the obstructive disease in the coronaries is the cause of the patient's chest pain or is suspected to be the cause.

- Specify/document whether the cause of the patient's documented cardiomyopathy is coronary occlusive disease (ischemic cardiomyopathy) or some other known cause (e.g., hypertension, valvular cardiomyopathy, viral cardiomyopathy, amyloid).

- Specify/document in the medical record of a patient with documented coronary artery bypass grafting (CABG) whether the symptoms are due to disease of the remaining native vessels or due to occlusion of bypass vein or artery or other graft. Identify the vessel or graft material, if known.

- Specify/document whether your patient has had angioplasty and a stent, and whether the current symptoms are due to occlusion of other native vessels or of the stent.

- Specify/document the cause if a patient with CAD developed unstable angina because of anemia or tachyarrhythmia or other secondary cause (demand ischemia causing unstable angina) and not new narrowing of the coronary arteries.

Debridement

Several treatment modalities are available for debridement. Debridement may be part of the cleaning of an open wound in preparation for closure, a comminuted fracture, or a burn in preparation for applying a skin graft. None of these requires specific documentation.

Within ICD classifications, **excisional debridement** is the excision of devitalized tissue, necrosis, and/or slough using sharp instruments (e.g., scissors, laser, or cutting curette) down to healthy tissue to enable speedier healing. It is imperative that providers document the deepest tissue actually removed (e.g., skin and subcutaneous tissue, tendon sheath, muscle, and/or bone).

Nonexcisional debridement includes cleaning out of debris or necrotic tissue of a wound with use of forceps, water jet, chemicals, or wet-to-dry dressings.

The diagnosis of the lesion(s) actually debrided is essential for proper classification (e.g., burn, infected surgical wound, pressure ulcer, arterial ulcer, venous stasis ulcer, diabetic neuropathic or vascular ulcer).

Documentation needs

- Identify/document the condition for which debridement is being performed (e.g., arterial ulcer, venous ulcer, neuropathic ulcer, pressure ulcer, open fracture, wound infection).

- Document whether the procedure is performed in the operating room or at the patient's bedside whenever the procedure was done sharply (with scissors or knife) to excise necrotic tissue from a wound, infection, or burn down to healthy granulation tissue.

- Document whether the procedure was merely to clean the edges of a laceration before closure.

- Document whether the procedure involved removing abraded, dirty tissue or bone fragments before closure or fixation of an open fracture.

- Clarify/document in the medical record whether the procedure was debridement of toenails to differentiate it from debridement of a foot ulcer, for example.

- Designate/document when a method other than excisional technique was used.

- Clarify/document the deepest tissue actually removed and the size of the area of the lesion debrided.

Dementia, Delirium, and Encephalopathy

Background

Altered mental status (time, place, and person) or **altered level of consciousness** (awake, unresponsive, comatose) can have multiple possible causes, some of which can be life-threatening and require immediate evaluation and initiation of treatment, and others with which patients will live the rest of their lives. The workup—and diagnosis after workup—is very important for poisonings or overdoses of narcotic, sedative, tranquilizer, or illicit drugs; septic metabolic encephalopathy; and senile dementia.

Definitions

Dementia is a long-term condition and is due to progressive destruction of brain cells. Dementia is a loss of brain function that occurs with certain diseases. It affects memory, thinking, language, judgment, and behavior. Most types of dementia are nonreversible (degenerative).[1]

1. Dementia, *diwanneurology.com/dementia.html*.

Alzheimer's disease is the most common type of dementia. Lewy body disease is a leading cause of dementia in elderly adults. People with this condition have abnormal protein structures in certain areas of the brain. Dementia also can be due to many small strokes. This is called vascular dementia. The following medical conditions also can lead to dementia:

- Parkinson's disease

- Multiple sclerosis

- Huntington's disease

- Pick's disease

- Progressive supranuclear palsy[2]

Delirium is a condition of acute onset and short duration that may be a manifestation of many conditions. When it is such a manifestation, it is a symptom and the cause should be determined. It may be a symptom of a transient encephalopathy, such as hypernatremic encephalopathy; it may be a symptom of change in location for a patient with Alzheimer's dementia who becomes delirious when no longer in a familiar surrounding; or it may be due to the effect of alcohol, anti-Parkinson drugs, steroids, or other medications. It requires specificity and should not be sought as a diagnosis. It is a manifestation of something else.

2. Ibid.

"**Encephalopathy** is a term for any diffuse disease of the brain that alters brain function or structure."[3] Correct use of the term specifically excludes traumatic causes that may lead to coma. "Encephalopathy may be caused by infectious agents (bacteria, viruses, or prions), metabolic or mitochondrial dysfunction, prolonged exposure to toxic elements (including solvents, drugs, radiation, paints, industrial chemicals, and certain metals), chronic progressive trauma, poor nutrition, or lack of oxygen or blood flow to the brain."[4] Common neurological symptoms are progressive loss of memory and cognitive ability, subtle personality changes, inability to concentrate, lethargy, and progressive loss of consciousness. Other neurological symptoms may include myoclonus (involuntary twitching of a muscle or group of muscles), nystagmus (rapid, involuntary eye movement), tremor, muscle atrophy and weakness, dementia, seizures, and loss of ability to swallow or speak.[5]

Encephalopathy is divided into three major groups:

1. Hypoxic encephalopathy

- Consequence of circulatory arrest or significant hypoxic respiratory event, such as suffocation

- Disorders associated with cardiac procedures (e.g., CABG, valve replacement, surgery on thoracic aorta where circulation

---

3. Encephalopathy, Toxic, *www.myelectronicmd.com/get_reference.php?Id=1059&condition=ENCEPHAL OPATHY%2C%20TOXIC&symname=E&typ=3*.

4. Ibid.

5. Encephalopathy, *www.ninds.nih.gov/disorders/encephalopathy/encephalopathy.htm*.

---

to the brain is purposely compromised as part of the procedure, percutaneous procedures where disruption of atheroma at the root of the aorta may embolize to the brain), rule out stroke

2. Metabolic encephalopathy

- Associated with sepsis

- Hepatic, uremic, hypernatremic, or hyponatremic encephalopathies

- Hypercalcemia or hypernatremic encephalopathy with significant brain dysfunction specifically caused by the electrolyte imbalance

3. Toxic encephalopathy

- Iatrogenic disorders (chemotherapy, steroid-induced, vaccine-induced, complication of transplant)

- Lead exposure, toxic solvents

Other named encephalopathies:

- Mitochondrial encephalopathy

- Glycine encephalopathy

- Hashimoto's encephalopathy

- Transmissible spongiform encephalopathy

- Neonatal hypoxemic ischemic encephalopathy

What is not encephalopathy:

- Intentional sedation from medication

- Being drunk or high on improper use of drugs

- Vasovagal syncope

- Transient cerebrovascular hypoperfusion

- Postictal state

- Stroke or transient ischemic attack (TIA)

- Progressive dementia (identify cause)

- Transient delirium in an elderly patient with chronic, degenerative brain disease due to unfamiliarity with surroundings while in the hospital

- Nonspecific changes on an EEG (some individuals profess that because *encephalo-* means "brain" and *-pathy* means "disease of", the term *encephalophathy* applies to every abnormal condition of the brain; it does not)

Be aware of stroke causing change in awareness, subdural bleed, head trauma, TIA, syncope due to transient hypoperfusion of the brain (as in bradycardia, vasovagal syncope), generalized hypoxemia (as in pulmonary embolism), or other specific causes, and link the presentation to the cause.

Documentation needs

- Clarify/document whether the patient's altered mental status is due to one of the conditions identified in the record (indicate which one) or document the cause, if known.

- Document the likely cause of a patient's delirium, which is often a symptom of something else, such as generalized cerebrovascular ischemia, Alzheimer's disease, or toxic effects of drugs. When you can identify the likely cause of a patient's presentation and decide to address treatment or care to that cause, document the relationship in the medical record.

- Document whether the presentation of altered mental status is likely due to an organic cause or a psychological cause. An elderly patient may also have psychological problems that supersede the decreased brain function from dementia. Clarify this information.

- Document whether you think infection, sepsis, dehydration, or specific organ failure is causing the delirium and whether it represents the specific encephalopathy. Be specific when clarifying the relationship between this process and the mental status change.

- Document the relationship of the mental status change to any other disease process.

Fractures

Background

The trauma leading to fracture of a bone can vary depending on the patient's bone health. Patients with bone diseases may suffer fractures with minimal trauma. **Osteoporosis** is the number one cause of such fractures in the United States. When a bone is fractured with inadequate trauma to have fractured a normal bone and the condition is known, the result is a **pathologic fracture and it should be documented in the medical record as such.**

For vertebrae, fractures may be classified as traumatic, due to fatigue or pathologic fracture.

The specific location of the fracture in long bones must be identified:

- Epiphysis (growth plate) dislocation without other fracture

- Proximal or distal end of the bone, identifying whether through the epiphysis additionally

- Shaft of the bone

Open fractures must be identified further using Gustilo (-Anderson) classification of open fractures under ICD-10-CM:

- **Type I:** The wound is smaller than 1 cm, clean, and generally caused by a fracture fragment that pierces the skin (i.e., inside-out injury). This is the result of low-energy trauma, caused by occurrences such as falls from a sitting or standing position.

- **Type II:** The wound is longer than 1 cm, not contaminated, and without major soft tissue damage or defect. This is also a low-energy injury.

- **Type III:** The wound is longer than 1 cm, with significant soft tissue disruption. The mechanism often involves high-energy trauma, resulting in a severely unstable fracture with varying degrees of fragmentation. Type III fractures are further divided as follows:

– "III A: Soft tissue coverage of the fractured bone is adequate.

– "III B: Extensive injury to or loss of soft tissue, with periosteal stripping and exposure of bone, massive contamination, and severe comminution of the fracture. After debridement and irrigation a local or free flap is necessary for coverage.

– "III C: Any open fracture that is associated with an arterial injury that must be repaired, regardless of the degree of soft tissue injury."[6]

Femur fractures

Repair of a fractured femur depends on the viability of the bony fragments and the location along the femur. Some fractures require no surgery because they are well aligned and the patient is not likely to walk because of concomitant disease or the patient is too sick to undergo surgery. Some patients who are at risk for aseptic necrosis of the head of the femur and who are immobile already may undergo removal of the head and neck of the femur with no reconstruction (Girdlestone procedure).

Fractures around the neck of the femur are classified as **pertrochanteric, intertrochanteric,** or **subtrochanteric.** Orthopedists will select a CPT® code for open treatment of such fractures, depending on which

6. Open Fractures: Classification. *www.rcsed.ac.uk/fellows/lvanrensburg/ classification/commonfiles/open.htm.*

portion of the neck of the femur was fractured. They are all open surgery codes. ICD classifies open surgery on the basis of whether and when a reduction was performed. An alternative surgical approach is to perform a total replacement of the femoral head if it is assumed that the arterial supply to the head of the femur will lead to aseptic necrosis.

Fractures of the shaft of the femur or **supracondylar fractures** are often treated with insertion of an intramedullary rod.

It is imperative to determine whether fracture reduction was performed and whether it was done before or after the skin incision.

Femoral fractures, regardless of whether the patient goes to the operating room, are occasionally associated with other conditions, such as anemia due to acute blood loss from the fracture site itself—which may or may not lead to anemia and may or may not require blood transfusion—and the occurrence of fatty pulmonary emboli from the fracture site or venous pulmonary emboli from the immobility.

Documentation needs

- Document in the operative/procedure note whether you reduced the fracture at all (impacted and in good alignment) and whether reduction was achieved prior to or after the incision.

- Document whether the patient lost enough blood from the fracture for the hematocrit to drop to a level consistent with anemia that would warrant follow-up, monitoring, or transfusion. This is not a complication of surgery; it is anemia due to acute blood loss from the fracture.

- Document other chronic, stable conditions that are under treatment, even if they are being followed by another physician while the patient is in the hospital.

- Document a diagnosis for any treatments instituted in the postoperative phase, such as acute urinary retention, atelectasis, or volume overload—don't simply treat a condition without identifying it. If the condition is due to an identifiable disease, make the link (e.g., acute urinary retention due to benign prostatic hyperplasia, atelectasis due to morbid obesity). Do not call it "postoperative urinary retention" or "postoperative atelectasis."

- Document whether the current visit is part of the expected initial treatment of the fracture, whether healing is delayed, or whether the patient has nonunion or malunion of the fracture.

Gastrointestinal Bleed

Gastrointestinal (GI) bleeds can be slow, chronic conditions or acute, hemorrhagic events. Acute GI bleed may be:

- Of low enough volume or rate of bleed to not cause hemodynamic instability—no specific documentation is needed

- Of enough volume change to lead to tachycardia and hypotension, but not enough to cause significant organ hypoperfusion—reflective of hypovolemia

- Of large volume with sufficient hypotension to cause organ damage—reflective of hemorrhagic shock

Initial identification of the potential site of the bleed can be surmised by the character of the bleed:

- Bright red blood through the anus is most frequently lower GI bleed

- Bright red blood in vomitus is most frequently rapid upper GI bleed

- Coffee-ground vomitus often signifies slower upper GI bleed

- Black blood in stool (melena) signifies that the blood originated above the duodenum (esophagus or stomach)

Be aware that bleeding gums, nosebleed, or another source not associated with the GI tract, as well as ingestion of bismuth subsalicylate or drinking blood, can cause heme-positive stool.

Link findings on endoscopy to the bleed, if possible. Sometimes, pathologic findings are visualized but may not be actively bleeding at the time of the procedure. However, the endoscopist might consider them the likely source of the bleed. If you cannot locate the source, it is more appropriate to identify whether it is thought to be an upper GI bleed or a lower GI bleed rather than just documenting "melena," "hematochezia," or "vomiting blood."

Be sure to evaluate the patient's hemoglobin and hematocrit upon admission and throughout the hospital stay. Identify whether anemia ever develops. Determining whether the patient was anemic on admission and stayed anemic (until transfused, if transfusion is necessary) is important. The anemia may be due to chronic blood loss or some other source of anemia. (Refer to the Anemia section.) If a significant drop in hemoglobin and hematocrit occurs, it is likely an acute bleed.

A patient may have multiple causes of anemia, such as anemia due to chronic kidney disease (or some other cause) and acute anemia (progressive drop in red blood count) due to acute GI blood loss.

Documentation needs

- Document whether you think that the patient's GI bleed is causing anemia. Document whether anemia is due to acute blood loss or due to chronic blood loss.

- Document whether you suspect that the cause is upper GI or lower GI until you have done studies to prove it. Remember that rectal bleeds originate in the rectum. If the bleed is melena or hematochezia, use these terms instead until you determine the source.

- Clarify/document in the record whether tests indicate a GI tract lesion and whether you think the lesion is the origin of a GI bleed.

- Specify/document in the record which lesion you think is the cause of the bleed if you discover two or more lesions during your workup.

- Specify/document that you don't know the cause of the GI bleed if your workup reveals several possible lesions or no lesions and you still do not know the possible etiology of the GI blood loss.

Heart Failure

Background

Heart failure can be an acute condition requiring acute medical attention or a chronic, background condition. Heart failure can involve the left side of the heart only, the right side of the heart only, or both sides. The traditionally known concept of congestive heart failure (CHF) is caused by left heart failure, with backup of fluid into the lungs. With right heart failure, there is backup into the legs with edema, the abdomen with ascites, the liver with chronic passive congestion or cardiac cirrhosis, and the veins overall with jugular venous distension.

Cardiomyopathy

Cardiomyopathy is defined as the disease process that can affect heart function but alone does not indicate dysfunction. (Some cardiologists erroneously equate cardiomyopathy with chronic systolic heart failure.) Chronic heart failure can have many causes, including ischemic cardiomyopathy, valvular heart disease (or valvular cardiomyopathy), hypertensive heart disease (or hypertensive cardiomyopathy), alcoholic cardiomyopathy, hypertrophic cardiomyopathy (with or without outflow obstruction), and amyloidosis of the heart. Just because a patient has a cardiomyopathy does not mean that there is heart failure.

Dysfunction

When the left ventricle does not work properly, there is dysfunction. Chronic dysfunction comes from modeling of the left ventricular wall either with stiffness and inability to fill adequately during diastole (diastolic dysfunction) or with dilatation causing weak contractions during systole (systolic dysfunction). Just because there is dysfunction does not mean that there is heart failure.

Chronic left heart failure

When a patient with a cardiomyopathy (any of the previously mentioned processes) and dysfunction of the left ventricle first develops symptoms of heart failure, the patient has chronic heart failure from that point forward (or until a heart transplant is performed).

Right heart failure

Dilation or hypertrophy of the right ventricle can occur because of all the same cardiomyopathies as in left heart failure, except for different valves (tricuspid and pulmonic) and a different source of hypertension (pulmonary hypertension, either primary or secondary to some other disease).

Remember that exacerbation of chronic right heart failure is not the same as acute cor pulmonale. This is a very rare condition and is generally found only in massive pulmonary embolism or acute respiratory distress syndrome (ARDS) in patients who require ventilator assistance and whose echocardiograms show acute dilation of the right ventricle.

Acute left heart failure

Usually, the actual mechanism is acute diastolic dysfunction with fluid overloading the lungs. This can occur as an exacerbation of a patient's chronic heart failure status or be an independent event with no background left heart failure. Conditions such as tachyarrhythmia (AF with RVR or supraventricular or ventricular tachycardia or accelerated hypertension) will cause acute diastolic heart failure without any chronic component present. Rare conditions may cause acute systolic heart failure, such as an acute ischemic event (coronary occlusive MI or demand MI), or Takotsubo syndrome. Most hospital admissions are for acute exacerbation (or decompensation) of chronic heart failure. Documentation of the chronic state drives the proper coding. Examples are exacerbation of chronic diastolic heart failure with LVH and normal EF, or decompensation of chronic systolic failure with dilated LV and EF lower than 40%.

Left ventricular echocardiogram or ventriculogram

When the left ventricle is thickened (left ventricular hypertrophy) or stiff and has a normal ejection fraction (usually in the range of 55%–70%) in the presence of documented heart failure, it probably signifies **chronic left ventricular diastolic failure.** When the left ventricle is dilated and has an EF lower than 40% with documented CHF, the condition is likely **chronic left ventricular systolic failure.**

Need to know

- Left ventricular failure or right ventricular failure, or both (biventricular)?

- If left ventricular failure, is the patient in acute CHF (and name the mechanism causing it), chronic heart failure (and name the causative cardiomyopathy), or decompensation of a chronic heart failure?

Classification of heart failure

- **New York Heart Association Classes 1–4:** Class 1 is preheart failure; Classes 2 and 3 justify insertion of a defibrillator when associated with systolic dysfunction; Class 4 is terminal end-stage heart failure.

- **American Heart Association Stages 1–4:** Stage 1 is cardiomy-opathy—there is a disease but no dysfunction. Stage 2 is dysfunc-tion—there is systolic or diastolic dysfunction or both, but the patient has never had symptoms. Stage 3 is chronic heart fail-ure—cardiomyopathy with dysfunction due to the cardiomyopa-thy and patient has had symptoms of heart failure. Stage 4 is end-stage heart failure (same as New York Heart Association Class 4). The American College of Cardiology recognizes that stages 3 and 4 represent codable chronic heart failure cases.

- **Left ventricular diastolic dysfunction is divided into Stages I–III:** Patients with no symptoms, only findings on echo, are not chronic heart failure patients. Stages II and III have symptoms and may represent chronic heart failure.

Documentation needs

- With the documentation of CHF, clarify whether you are discussing right heart failure or left heart failure. If left heart failure, clarify whether this represents an acute or chronic state or both (provide BNP level for validation, if appropriate).

- Document the etiology of the cardiomyopathy (hypertensive heart disease, ischemic heart disease, valvular and which valve[s], viral, alcoholic).

- Document known results of cardiac function studies and indicate whether they reflect failure due to left ventricular systolic dysfunction, left ventricular diastolic dysfunction, or both.

- Clarify the patient's heart failure status (due to chronic left ventricular systolic or diastolic dysfunction) and whether the current episode reflects acute decompensation (e.g., "patient with chronic diastolic failure due to hypertensive heart disease with acute systolic decompensation due to non-Q wave MI").

- Document whether the patient had an acute MI within eight weeks of this episode and whether the acute MI caused this episode of decompensation. (Note that this will change to four weeks with ICD-10.)

- Identify/document the relationship if this patient has chronic renal failure (CRF) and if volume overload or noncardiac pulmonary edema led to the decompensation of CHF.

Hyperglycemia

Elevated blood sugar can occur in many conditions and does not automatically mean that the patient has diabetes or that a patient with known diabetes has uncontrolled diabetes. Treatment with insulin around the time of illness or surgery does not signify uncontrolled diabetes.

Patients with diabetes can develop elevated blood sugar with use of steroids for another condition, such as COPD or allergy, with infection, and with stress. Uncontrolled diabetes usually implies long-term lack of control and can be measured with glycosylated hemoglobin, or hemoglobin A1C, higher than 7.0 or difficulty in maintaining a job, good grades in school, or psychological balance over a long period of time.

Diabetes mellitus has four major classifications:

- **Type 1**—Patient was born with or acquired inability to produce insulin and cannot live without insulin

- **Type 2**—Patient acquired resistance to effects of insulin; may be diet controlled, on oral hypoglycemics, or may take insulin for added control

- **Secondary causes of diabetes**—Due to genetic disorder or poisoning of the islet cells or long-term use of steroids or after pancreatic surgery (see *www.hcpro.com/HIM-223721-147/ Go-back-to-the-source-when-coding-secondary-diabetes.html*)

- **Gestational diabetes**—Diabetes during pregnancy that resolves after delivery

Diabetic ketoacidosis or diabetic hyperosmolar coma can occur with extremely high levels of sugar. Ketoacidosis most frequently occurs in Type 1 diabetics, whereas non-ketotic acidosis or coma occurs in Type 2 diabetics.

Diabetes can have adverse effects on target organs:

- Diabetic retinopathy (proliferative or nonproliferative and stratified as mild, moderate, or severe, with or without macular edema)

- Diabetic nephropathy (stage 1–5 or ESRD)

- Diabetic autonomic neuropathy (specify with gastroparesis or Charcot foot or skin ulcer)

- Diabetic dermopathy—discolorations without serious side effects

- Diabetic skin ulcer (requires specificity if neuropathic ulcer, vascular ulcer, or due to progressive dermatitis of diabetes)

- Diabetic microvascular disease—can lead to gangrene of distal extremities, cerebral ischemia, heart ischemic

- Diabetic periodontal disease or other oral complications

Documentation needs

- Document whether the patient has diabetes. Indicate when it is uncontrolled. Although hemoglobin A1C determination may be helpful, your clinical impression is just as important.

- Document whether the patient has type 1 (i.e., does not make insulin), type 2 (i.e., is resistant to insulin), or other secondary cause of diabetes. If this patient has adult-onset diabetes and is taking insulin, document "type 2, taking insulin," and not "insulin dependent" (avoid using the terms *IDDM* and *NIDDM*).

- Distinguish between uncontrolled diabetes and situational hyperglycemia in a diabetic patient along with the cause of the hyperglycemia (e.g., steroid-induced hyperglycemia in a controlled Type 2 diabetic or stress-induced hyperglycemia).

- Identify/document the infectious source if this episode of hyperglycemia was precipitated by an infection. If this incident represents sepsis from a source, identify/document it as "sepsis due to ..." If related to an indwelling device (e.g., cardiac valve, Foley catheter, vascular access device), identify the device as the source.

- Document whether the patient has other manifestations of diabetes (e.g., gastroparesis, diabetic renal failure, blindness, neuropathy).

- Identify/document the reason for hyperglycemia (e.g., steroid therapy, other endocrine dysfunction) if this patient is not diabetic.

Hypertension

Background

Elevation of systemic blood pressure can be a situational condition and either transient or chronic. Either can be dangerous to patients. ICD codes for hypertension presume the chronic disease, and extensions of the code sets relate to the target organs that may be affected by hypertension. Target organs of both the acute and chronic varieties are the brain, the kidneys, and the heart.

Figure 1 illustrates the chronic and acute ways that hypertension affects target organs.

Figure 1: Target Organs for Hypertension

	Chronic	Acute
Brain	Ischemic brain disease with white matter shrinkage and vascular dementia	Hypertensive encephalopathy Hypertensive seizure Hypertensive stroke
Kidneys	Chronic kidney disease	Acute kidney injury
Heart	Hypertensive heart disease with left ventricular hypertrophy (dilates in end-stage HHD) and chronic diastolic heart failure	Acute pulmonary edema Acute diastolic heart failure Unstable angina Acute NSTEMI

Source: Robert S. Gold, MD.

In adults, hypertension and diabetes are the two most common causes of chronic kidney disease, whereas in children, chronic kidney disease is one of the most common causes of hypertension.

Hypertensive emergency is defined as accelerated or malignant hypertension (i.e., blood pressure in the range of 220/140) with acute target organ damage, whereas hypertensive urgency is accelerated or malignant hypertension without acute target organ damage.

Documentation needs

- Distinguish whether elevated blood pressure signifies a transient condition due to another disease or condition or represents systemic essential hypertension.

- Clarify whether documented hypertensive emergency or hypertensive crisis represents accelerated or malignant essential hypertension, hypertension due to renal artery stenosis, hypertension due to endocrine disorder (e.g., pheochromocytoma, thyrotoxicosis), or hypertension due to some other cause.

- Clarify/document the use of the term *hypertensive emergency* in the absence of identified acute target organ damage. Is it hypertensive urgency?

- Clarify/document the use of the term *hypertensive urgency* if there is documentation of target organ damage. Is it hypertensive emergency?

- With documentation of kidney disease and chronic hypertension, clarify which is the causative factor—hypertension causing chronic kidney disease (CKD) or specific chronic kidney disease leading to hypertension. Clarify the stage of CKD.

Inflammatory Bowel Disease

Background

Physicians take several shortcuts when describing patients with intestinal disorders, such as documenting IBD, which can be interpreted as either irritable bowel disease or inflammatory bowel disease, and IBS, which is often irritable bowel syndrome.

Irritable bowel describes a condition generally with hypermotility of the intestines associated with abdominal cramping and diarrhea. This is a nonspecific term and is often used as a means to classify a patient either until general medical treatment is effective or to justify more tests, such as abdominal x-rays, CT, MRI, or endoscopy. It can be caused by psychologic issues, spasm of the intestinal muscles associated with development of diverticular disease, or ischemia of the intestinal tract, or it can be descriptive of inflammatory bowel disease. The specific cause of irritable bowel should be sought, and, if it can be identified, specific therapy can be provided. Otherwise, general medical and or psychologic treatments may be provided if and until the specific cause is identified.

Inflammatory bowel disease has two major components—Crohn's disease and ulcerative colitis. Some cases are identified with elements of both.

Crohn's disease (sometimes referred to as terminal ileitis) has some genetic predisposition and may have minimal to devastating manifestations. It may be identified in virtually any area of the intestinal tract (i.e., duodenum, jejunum, ileum, colon, rectum) or in multiple areas of the intestinal tract and may have skip areas of normal bowel in between inflamed segments.

Ulcerative colitis similarly has some genetic predisposition and is associated with development of colon cancer after a number of years with the disease. It generally starts in the colorectal area of the large intestine and progresses proximally, involving left colon, transverse colon, right colon, and cecum, with no skip areas.

Documentation needs

Clarify and document the following only if the clinical picture seems appropriate:

- The abbreviation you used as meaning inflammatory bowel or irritable bowel disease or syndrome. If inflammatory, indicate whether the patient has Crohn's disease or ulcerative colitis.

- Crohn's disease and ulcerative colitis may be defined by area of the bowel involved. Specify/document which areas of the intestinal tract are involved. For Crohn's disease, identify/document the specific area involved (i.e., terminal ileum, duodenum, colon, multiple areas with skip lesions). For ulcerative colitis, identify how proximally the disease has progressed.

- Specific complications of Crohn's disease or ulcerative colitis should be identified and tracked when appropriate. Identify/document whether the patient has the following:

  - Bleeding (acute bleeding or chronic bleeding, and whether it has caused anemia)

  - Perforation with or without abscess, and the location of the abscess

  - Obstruction

  - Fistula

Low Anterior Resection

Cancers of the large intestine are classified, for the purposes of the tumor registry and other tracking, by the location of the cancer in the bowel. Treatment of these cancers is similarly classified by the portion of the intestine removed. Surgeons use CPT® codes to bill for their procedures. For most surgeries performed, they use one particular CPT code for "partial resection of colon with low pelvic anastomosis." This definition may lead some physicians astray in describing the operation they performed from the perspective of ICD-10-PCS coding.

Low anterior resection is an operation designed for resection of a cancer in the midportion of the rectum with end-to-end anastomosis. If end-to-end anastomosis is impossible for these rectal cancers, an abdominoperineal resection is the alternative.

Other colon resections for colon cancers include right hemicolectomy, left hemicolectomy, sigmoidectomy, total abdominal colectomy, and other resections (e.g., resection of the transverse colon for cancers located in the midportion of the transverse colon).

Other pathologic conditions may lead to similar operative procedures, such as diverticulitis, multiple polyposis, and ulcerative colitis. For proper ICD-10-PCS coding, the portion of the intestine where the pathologic condition is located, the name of the pathologic condition, and the portion of the large intestine actually removed are necessary.

Documentation needs

- Define and document in the medical record whether the disease process originated in the sigmoid colon, in the rectum, or at the rectosigmoid junction.

- Clarify/document whether the disease was of the sigmoid colon or rectum in resections for diverticular disease. *Sigmoidectomy* would be the appropriate term if sigmoid disease and not low anterior resection, which implies that only the rectum was resected.

- Specify/document which part of the bowel was resected (e.g., sigmoidectomy, rectal resection) and if there is cancer or a premalignant lesion, such as villous adenoma. The tumor registry collects data based on location of a malignancy and the part of bowel removed even though physicians bill resection with or without colostomy or with low pelvic anastomosis. Specifying/ documenting this information makes the data more valuable.

Note: In cases of anemia due to chronic blood loss from the lesion (diverticular bleed or malignant lesion bleed), specify/document that the anemia was due to chronic blood loss from the lesion.

Malignancies

Neoplasms, or tumors, may involve almost any tissue. They may be **benign, malignant,** or **indeterminant** by pathologic examination. The malignancies may be localized within an organ, may have spread from the original location but still within the organ, may have spread to other tissues adjacent to and outside of the organ, or may have metastasized to regional lymph nodes or through the bloodstream to other organs, such as the liver, lungs, or brain.

The following is required for proper determination of a patient's current status:

- The name of the primary tumor if the primary tumor is present.

- Whether it is benign or malignant.

- Whether it has spread to other tissues regionally.

- Whether it has spread to lymph nodes.

- Whether it has spread to other organs and which specific organs.

- If the primary tumor has been removed and the patient is admitted for treatment for metastatic disease, each organ in which metastatic disease is identified must be identified (principal diagnosis is the metastatic site).

- Whether the patient is admitted for workup and identification of the original diagnosis is made on this admission or the patient is admitted for radiotherapy or chemotherapy with the diagnosis having already been made.

- Whether the patient is admitted only for treatment of a manifestation of the tumor, such as anemia or malnutrition.

- Whether the patient is admitted for pain control with no treatment directed at the cancer.

- Whether the patient with terminal disease is converted to comfort measures only with no further treatment provided other than comfort care.

- Whether the patient is admitted with terminal cancer and no diagnosis has been made pathologically but all tests signify that it is undoubtedly cancer. If the physician is sure this is the problem, code this as though the cancer diagnosis has been made.

Documentation needs

- Identify/document the primary source of the malignancy and indicate whether that primary source is still being treated or has been treated and is no longer present. Do not use the term *history of* if the malignancy is still present. Use this term only if the primary source is completely gone.

- Identify/document whether there is a recurrence at the same site or a reappearance elsewhere (i.e., metastasis) and to which site.

- Clarify/document the organ of metastasis to distinguish from the organ of origin ("lung met" could be interpreted as either metastasis of testicular cancer to the lung or metastasis of lung cancer to the brain, unless you are specific).

- Clarify/document whether current symptoms are related to direct invasion of the malignancy, related to the pressure effect, or completely unrelated to the presence of the malignancy.

- Document a malignancy as a malignancy if a scan or x-ray confirms it. "Mass" is not "cancer." "Tumor" is not "cancer." Biopsy confirmation is not necessary to call it a cancer if you truly believe it is a malignancy.

- In documentation of leukemias, clarify whether the visit involves leukemia in remission, leukemia cured, or leukemia never having (yet) achieved remission. "History of" does not tell the story.

Malnutrition

Background

Malnutrition has adverse effects on the body's ability to defend itself against invading microorganisms, to heal after surgery or trauma, and to maintain homeostasis during any hospital intervention. Although seen more in the elderly, different specific types of malnutrition can also occur in the pediatric population.

Malnutrition can be due to inadequate intake of proteins, fats, and sugars as well as vitamins, minerals, and other substances that the body requires to perform daily functions. Many conditions caused by the lack of vitamin and mineral intake have their own specific names (e.g., iron deficiency anemia, scurvy, pellagra) and are not discussed in this book.

In many disease states, malnutrition is an inherent risk factor, and preventive treatments are often provided to prevent malnutrition. An example is short gut syndrome, for which a patient may receive nutritional supplements or intravenous hyperalimentation to maintain good nutritional status. Most patients with cirrhosis, terminal malignancies, or renal failure or who receive high-powered antimetabolites and chemotherapeutic drugs (as in cancer therapy) are constantly malnourished.

For tracking purposes, malnutrition has been stratified as mild, moderate, and severe. When protein stores are severely depleted, whether acutely or chronically, protein energy malnutrition (previously called protein calorie malnutrition) occurs.

Patients who are severely protein depleted may be edematous because of the lack of protein to maintain intravascular oncotic pressure, but they may appear healthy. Other patients may appear cachectic or wasted. Defining and stratifying the level of malnutrition in these patients is important. The terms *kwashiorkor* and *marasmus* are not typically used in the United States, but these patients also have protein malnutrition. These specific terms are not necessary to determine that a patient has protein calorie malnutrition or to stratify the level as mild, moderate, or severe.

Many screening tools exist for determination of this severity; they are often called **subjective global assessments** of nutrition. The physician's ability to look at a patient and the patient's history may be all that is necessary to determine that a patient is severely malnourished. The American Society for Parenteral and Enteral Nutrition (ASPEN) has developed current standards in the dietary world, and a hospital's nutritional support team should be aware of its risk stratification techniques.

Levels of protein alone, of albumin alone, or of prealbumin are inadequate to determine the presence, much less the level, of malnutrition. Addition of such evaluations as patient's body mass index (BMI) or percentage of loss in body weight (specifically not loss in water weight, as can occur with diuretics, removal of ascites, or delivery of a baby) can make a difference. Most authorities will recognize that unplanned loss of body mass less than 10% represents mild malnutrition, between 10% and 20% is consistent with moderate malnutrition, and more than 20% implies severe malnutrition.

Malnutrition evaluation in children has specific guidelines as related to expected levels of growth and development. Several methodologies are used that compare weight-to-height ratios, weight-for-age ratios, BMI, and deviation from expected and other techniques.

Malnutrition in a newborn is often related to problems with the mother and her nutritional habits. Review of the dietary notes can be helpful.

In addition to the presence of malnutrition stratified by severity, identifying the cause of malnutrition is clinically pertinent:

- Acute malnutrition due to complex trauma or extensive surgery

- Acute malnutrition due to acute disease, such as acute ischemic bowel disease, clostridia enterocolitis, necrotizing pancreatitis, or sepsis

- Chronic malnutrition due to chronic disease, such as Crohn's disease, short bowel syndrome, chronic ischemic bowel disease, or cancer

- Chronic malnutrition due to child or elder abuse by not feeding the individual

- Chronic malnutrition due to psychological disorder, such as bulimia, other psychological disease

A morbidly obese person can be severely malnourished. Malnutrition should also be considered in psychological disturbances, including binging/purging manifestations, as can occur with bulimia. Documentation in the medical record of the specific type and degree of malnutrition will be valuable to patient care and outcomes.

Documentation needs

- The patient's loss of pounds over the past months has been identified. This translates to a percentage loss in body mass.

- The patient's BMI has been identified as ____%, and there is an order for dietary supplementation. Identification of malnourished state and stratifying its severity is important in determining increased risk to healing.

- Please help identify whether the patient's nutritional status is depleted and stratify the level of malnutrition (i.e., mild, moderate, severe), if appropriate. (Provide the documented clinical evidence to support the need for this question.)

Note: The terms *cachexia* or *wasted appearance* are identified by most physicians at the time of admission. Identification of the cause of this appearance may be beneficial in stratifying the patient's risk.

Regulatory bodies have closely monitored and audited malnutrition documentation during the past several years. Physicians and health information management staff must work closely together on improvement activities and general awareness of the documentation of specific types of malnutrition.

Obesity

Obesity poses a serious risk to a satisfactory outcome in the hospital. Physical and metabolic aspects of the obese patient can lead to the need for hospitalization. Obese patients have a higher risk of complications from anesthesia and surgery, and concomitant malnutrition that can occur in these patients can hinder resistance to infection.

Obesity is stratified grossly as obese and **morbidly obese,** with the latter defined as 100 pounds over ideal body weight, or a BMI of 40 or higher. Most morbidly obese patients will develop secondary diseases such as the following:

- Type 2 diabetes

- Hypertension with left ventricular strain causing left ventricular hypertrophy and diastolic dysfunction

- Gastroesophageal reflux

- Cellulitis under the folds of the pannus or under the arms

- Osteoarthrosis of the joints of the leg, leading to need for joint replacement surgery

Documentation of these secondary diseases should appear in the medical record so that they can be coded.

People living with a large abdominal size for long periods of time may develop **obesity hypoventilation syndrome (Pickwickian syndrome),** with pressure from the abdomen resulting in the following:

- Sleep apnea (often related to nocturnal regurgitation from gastroesophageal reflux).

- Restriction of the movement of the diaphragm with respiration leading to secondary pulmonary hypertension from the restrictive lung disease. This leads to the following:

  - Right heart strain

- Chronic cor pulmonale; this condition is accompanied by increased venous pressure in the right atrium, which then leads to the following:

  - Chronic passive congestion of the liver or cardiac cirrhosis

  - Ascites

  - Deep venous disease in the legs

  - Secondary hypercoagulable state

  - Edema of the legs with cellulitis

All of these should be documented when they exist, as they may individually or as a group lead to in-hospital morbidity and mortality.

Documentation needs

- Clarify/document whether your patient identified as overweight is, indeed, obese. BMI has been determined to be _____.

- Identify/document patients who are morbidly obese, because this carries a significant impact in morbidity and mortality outcomes for hospitalization.

- Identification of patients with morbid obesity is important with respect to tracking the secondary conditions associated with morbid obesity (e.g., type 2 diabetes, hypertension, gastroesophageal reflux with its risk of aspiration pneumonitis, osteoarthrosis of hips and knees).

- Identification of patients with obesity hypoventilation syndrome (morbid obesity plus secondary pulmonary artery hypertension) is important because of the added risk of morbidity and mortality associated with this condition (e.g., restrictive lung disease, cor pulmonale, congestive liver disease from cardiac cirrhosis, secondary hypercoagulable state). Identify each of the problems your patient demonstrates from obesity hypoventilation syndrome.

Peripheral Vascular Disease

Background

Circulatory disease can involve the peripheral circulation; distinguishing between peripheral arterial disease (PAD) and peripheral venous disease (PVD) is most important. There are varying severities of both, and each deserves proper, documented attention.

Peripheral arterial disease

Identify the disease condition. It can involve atherosclerosis, immunologic conditions, neurological causes, or external causes of decreased circulation to the extremities. Documenting the following is important:

- Identify the blood vessel of concern by its position in the extremity (proximal, distal, thigh, leg, foot, toes) or the specific blood vessel involved (superficial femoral, dorsalis pedis, brachial artery)

- Indicate whether it was chronic narrowing or embolic (and the source of the embolism)

- Enumerate presence of manifestations, such as claudication, rest pain, ulceration, or gangrene

Peripheral venous disease

Identify the disease condition. Identify the part of the extremity involved (thigh, calf, ankle, part of foot) or the specific vein(s) (superficial or deep veins, femoral, popliteal, sural veins, etc.), and manifestations (ulceration, pain, swelling).

Documentation of the specific peripheral disease will help the coding process capture the data to reflect a patient's disease state and the appropriate level of accuracy.

Pneumonia

Pneumonias are classified by the organism causing the infection, if known, or by three other entities: **aspiration pneumonitis** (which includes aspiration pneumonia), **empyema** (infected pleural effusion or pyothorax), and **lung abscess.**

Loeffler's syndrome, also known as **eosinophilic pneumonia,** is an allergic phenomenon.

Hypostatic pneumonia is a postmortem finding; no patients are admitted for treatment of hypostatic pneumonia. The term originated to depict settling of blood in the lungs from long-term (months to years) immobility and occurs in the end stages of terminal illness. Do not encourage use of this term.

Pneumonitis is a chemical inflammation of the lungs that can be caused by aspiration of gastric acid or other toxic chemicals. It can be followed by true pneumonia because of the setting up of irritated areas in the lung that will be prone to secondary infection and can lead to acute respiratory distress syndrome (ARDS).

Aspiration pneumonitis, aspiration pneumonia, and **aspiration bronchitis** are defined, for the purposes of ICD-10-CM coding, as related to aspiration of foodstuffs or gastric content that can lead to acute pulmonary edema and ARDS with acute respiratory failure, persistent coughing and wheezing, or an indolent infection in an elderly patient. It is not to be mistaken for the mode of transmission of bacteria into the lungs from a patient's mouth or through droplet transmission from another person.

Hospital core measures guidelines for pneumonia patients include administration of appropriate antibiotics within two hours of diagnosis. To this end, patients at high risk of aspiration pneumonia or *Pseudomonas* pneumonia or any other identifiable organism through culture or history should have antibiotic regimens prepared for these organisms. The physician should evaluate all pneumonia admissions for these contingencies.

Pneumonia is a clinical diagnosis, and pneumonias can be diagnosed with normal chest x-rays if the clinical findings and physical examination convince the physician. If an initial thought of pneumonia is made in the emergency department but further notes regarding the patient no longer mention pneumonia, clarify whether it was ruled out as a valid diagnosis.

Ventilator-associated pneumonia is pneumonia that develops after a patient has been on a ventilator for a period of time; it does not identify a patient admitted with pneumonia who requires a ventilator for acute respiratory failure.

Documentation needs

- Evaluate the patient's identified risk of aspiration as the cause of the pneumonia from the perspectives of debilitating gastroesophageal reflux disease (GERD), alcoholism, bed-ridden status, and pharyngeal dysfunction. Document whether you believe that there is a link between the patient's dysphagia or GERD and the identified pneumonia. Clarify whether this is aspiration pneumonia or aspiration pneumonitis, as appropriate.

- Clarify/document whether the infiltrate identified in your notes from the chest x-ray likely represents pneumonia, CHF, chronic lung disease, ARDS, Loeffler's syndrome, atelectasis, or lung cancer.

- Document in the medical record whether you are using antibiotics to treat specific organisms that you believe are the likely cause of pneumonia (e.g., *Klebsiella, Pseudomonas, Streptococcus,* methicillin-resistant *Staphylococcus aureus,* methicillin-sensitive *Staphylococcus aureus,* aerobic Gram-negative rods) even in the absence of positive sputum culture. **Do not identify a pneumonia as *possible Gram-negative pneumonia* or other similar term if you intend to use broad-spectrum coverage and have no idea what the causative organism is.**

- Identify/document patients admitted with pneumonia that started with specific influenza virus infections (e.g., novel swine influenza, avian influenza) to distinguish them from a patient who has pneumonia and an incidental positive test for specific influenza viruses, unrelated to the pneumonia. Identify superinfections by cultured organisms. Distinguish from viral pneumonia caused by the influenza organism.

- If you believe that a case represents pneumonia, despite a normal chest x-ray in a patient who is dehydrated or otherwise does not demonstrate an infiltrate, clarify it in the medical record documentation.

- Link organisms found in sputum or blood culture to the pneumonia if you believe they are the causative organisms.

Regulatory attention to pneumonia documentation or lack thereof has been greater in the past. A good understanding of documentation needs can help protect a hospital, organization, or practice against regulatory audits and reviews.

Pulmonary Edema

Background

Fluid in the interstitial spaces in the lung or fluid in the alveoli can be interpreted as **pulmonary edema.** With severe shortness of breath, it is likely **acute pulmonary edema.** Chronic pulmonary edema is usually a manifestation of end-stage heart failure. Patients with acute pulmonary edema may present with acute respiratory failure. Identifying acuity and cause in the clinical documentation is important.

Cardiac causes of acute pulmonary edema include:

- Exacerbation of left ventricular heart failure, including with volume overload in end stage renal disease (ESRD) patients who have chronic heart failure

- Acute MI, whether from coronary occlusion or demand MI

- Accelerated (or malignant) hypertension, including the severe hypertension that may occur with thyrotoxicosis, pheochromocytoma, carcinoid syndrome, eclampsia

- Tachyarrhythmia (AF with RVR, supraventricular tachycardia, ventricular tachycardia)

- Takotsubo syndrome (stress cardiomyopathy or apical ballooning syndrome)

Noncardiac causes of acute pulmonary edema include:

- Pulmonary embolism (venous thrombi, fat or air embolism)

- Aspiration of gastric acid

- Aspiration of toxic fumes and vapors

- Sepsis (acute respiratory distress syndrome [ARDS])

- Rapid decompression

- Drowning

- Volume overload in ESRD patients who do not have chronic heart failure

Documentation needs

- If this was an acute MI (including non-Q wave MI due to ventricular tachycardia, pulmonary embolism, or fat embolus), document it as the cause of the acute pulmonary edema.

- If there was chest trauma, rapid deceleration, sepsis, or ARDS, document it as the cause of the acute pulmonary edema.

- If the patient aspirated fumes, vapors, gastric acid, or food, document it as the cause of the acute pulmonary edema.

- If this volume overload is related to renal failure with an otherwise stable heart, document it as noncardiac acute pulmonary edema. Document when an ESRD patient has heart failure due to volume overload. *Example:* "Noncompliant patient missed dialysis two days ago, admitted now in volume overload causing exacerbation of chronic diastolic heart failure."

Renal Failure

As with other diseased organs, kidneys and renal function can undergo chronic changes (chronic kidney disease [CKD]) as well as acute changes. **Acute renal failure** (ARF) or acute kidney injury can be of varying severity, result from various causes, and lead to total resolution or residual deficit in renal functional capabilities.

CKD has myriad causes, with diabetes and hypertension the most frequent in the United States. Decreases in renal function can progress very slowly or very rapidly. The National Kidney Foundation™ supports following a patient's **glomerular filtration rate** (GFR) to determine whether there is change, and if there is decrease in function, taking measures to control the disease that has caused that decrease in function. If progress is rapid, the patient must be prepared for dialysis or transplantation, if clinically appropriate.

CKD is staged according to GFR with formulas designed for infants and children (Schwartz equation) and for adults up to age 83 (Fadem equation). Figure 2 illustrates the five recognized stages of progressive severity.

Figure 2: Five Stages Severity Chart

Stage	Severity	GFR
1	Kidney damage with normal or raised GFR	> 90 ml/min/1.73m²
2	Kidney damage with mild decrease GFR	60–90 ml/min/1.73m²
3	Moderate decrease in GFR	30–59 ml/min/1.73m²
4	Severe decrease in GFR	15–29 ml/min/1.73m²
5	Kidney failure GFR	< 15 ml/min/1.73m²

Source: Robert S. Gold, MD.

Stage 5 CKD is considered kidney failure and, depending on the clinical situation, may require dialysis. Not all Stage 5 CKD patients undergo dialysis, so they should not be referred to as having ESRD. When a patient with Stage 4 or 5 CKD has been on chronic dialysis for three months, the patient is considered ESRD for billing purposes.

Acute renal failure can occur as a result of many causes, the most common of which is severe dehydration. Due to toxicity from acetaminophen or from iodide dyes used for contrast radiography or aminoglycosides (gentamicin, tobramycin, amikacin), efforts must be made to avoid kidney injury when these drugs are given. Treatment of acute renal failure ranges from rehydration to acute need for dialysis.

Fractional excretion of sodium (FeNa) may be useful in identifying acute tubular necrosis as the mechanism of the acute renal failure along with identification of tubular casts in the urinalysis.

Changes in creatinine level or urine output may define the three stages of acute renal failure (acute kidney injury [AKI]). A person who is dehydrated should not be identified as having suffered from acute renal failure until having been resuscitated for at least six hours. If creatinine levels return to predehydration level in about that time interval, the patient was merely dehydrated. Distinction must be made between elevated creatinine level due to hemoconcentration and AKI, which does not immediately respond to fluid challenge. Figure 3 illustrates the stages of acute kidney injury.

Figure 3: AKI Stages Chart

AKI stage	Creatinine criteria	Urine output criteria
AKI stage I	Increase of serum creatinine by >/= 0.3 mg/dl (>/= 26.4 umol/L) or increase to >/= 150% – 200% from baseline	Urine output < 0.5 ml/kg/hour for > 6 hours
AKI stage II	Increase of serum creatinine to > 200% – 300% from baseline	Urine output < 0.5 ml/kg/hour for > 12 hours
AKI stage III	Increase of serum creatinine to > 300% from baseline or (>/= 354 ?mol/L) after a rise of at least 44 umol/L or treatment with renal replacement therapy	Urine output < 0.3 ml/kg/hour for > 24 hours or anuria for 12 hour

Documentation needs

- Recognize that acute renal insufficiency is not the same as acute renal failure or acute kidney injury. If the creatinine rises 0.3 mg higher than the patient's normal level, this is consistent with failure or AKI. If due to dehydration and the patient's creatinine returns to baseline within six hours, AKI did not likely occur, but the changes in creatinine only represent hemoconcentration.

- Document the cause of the acute renal failure/acute kidney injury (e.g., severe dehydration, sepsis, rhabdomyolysis, obstruction).

- Identify the pathologic mechanism of the acute renal failure/ acute kidney injury when known (e.g., acute tubular necrosis, acute medullary necrosis, acute cortical necrosis).

- Determine the stage of CKD in all patients with previously documented chronic renal insufficiency (CRI) or chronic renal failure (CRF). Documenting the stages will determine severity of illness. Although CRI or CRF is now useless for that determination, you should still use the phrase ESRD when the patient has been on chronic dialysis (three months).

- Use the GFR calculator (MDRD or Cockroft, or for children and infants, Schwartz formula) to determine GFR and convert it to the appropriate CKD stage. Document it in inpatient or outpatient medical records. The complexity of medical decision-making also depends on this information.

Note: When a patient has CKD, regardless of stage, document the cause of the renal disease in the patient's medical record (e.g., hypertension, diabetes, chronic pyelonephritis, lupus nephritis, myeloma).

Respiratory Failure

Background

Delivery of oxygen to the body and elimination of carbon dioxide is the goal of respiration. When anything that significantly impairs the processes to meet that goal occurs, the patient is in respiratory failure (unless the patient is purposely anesthetized or sedated and being maintained on a ventilator to avoid respiratory failure).

Many conditions can block delivery of oxygen or impede the clearance of carbon dioxide, or both. **Hypoxemic respiratory failure** is referred to as **type 1 respiratory failure; ventilatory failure** or **hypercapnic**

respiratory failure is referred to as **type 2.** However, documenting only the type will not lead to proper ICD-10 code assignment.

Chronic

Patients may be in a chronic state of respiratory failure due to musculoskeletal diseases (e.g., polio or cervical spine injury with paralysis of respiratory muscles), alveolar damage (e.g., pulmonary fibrosis, emphysema), or obstructive airways (e.g., COPD, bronchiectasis, cystic fibrosis). These patients demonstrate hypoxemia with PaO_2 under 55 on room air or compensated respiratory acidosis with hypercapnia with either pH = 7.4 and pCO_2 over 50 or HCO_3 on basic metabolic panel over 30 (in the absence of other acid-base imbalance).

Acute

Patients may present with acute respiratory failure due to many causes:

- Musculoskeletal in origin, as with acute spinal injury

- Viral infections that lead to paralysis (e.g., Guillain-Barre syndrome)

- Overdoses of narcotic or illicit drugs; severe hypoxemia due to pulmonary embolism (whether venous, fat, or air in origin)

- Damage to the lung tissue, as with inhalation of acid, alkaline fumes, or gastric acid

- Loss of functional lung tissue, as in severe atelectasis; pneumothorax or pleural effusion

- ARDS from numerous possible causes

- Obstruction from acute exacerbations of COPD from pneumonia or bronchitis or unknown cause

- Exacerbations of cystic fibrosis

- A foreign body

These patients will have acute distress in breathing, often using accessory muscles of respiration (neck muscles, abdominal breathing), breathing rapidly (more than 28 breaths per minute), being unable to speak more than two-word sentences, or exhibiting peripheral cyanosis. They may respond rapidly to interventional drugs or other specific treatments and, by the time they arrive in the nursing unit, no longer demonstrate any of these symptoms, but the circumstances of admission certainly included acute respiratory failure. A patient may demonstrate hypoxia or compensated respiratory acidosis but not be sick enough to call it acute respiratory failure. Call it what it is.

What is not acute respiratory failure?

- Some patients will be intubated and placed on a ventilator for protective reasons when there is not (yet) acute respiratory failure, such as patients who have had a significant stroke or who have laryngeal angioedema due to allergic reaction or patients with swelling of the neck in trauma

- Patients may be intubated after stroke or traumatic brain injury when there is risk that they may not be able to protect their own airways

- Patients electively being maintained on a ventilator overnight after surgery only to be weaned the next day when there is a full team available do not have acute respiratory failure

- Patients who have planned a return to the operating room for either a staged procedure or to evaluate intestinal viability or assumption of transplant liver function

- Children who have undergone surgery for congenital heart disease will usually be maintained on a ventilator for one to two days postoperatively to minimize stresses on the circulatory system while the heart is adjusting to the new circulatory pattern

Documentation needs

- Document in the medical record whether you believe that the patient has respiratory failure in addition to any other diagnoses.

- Document whether the respiratory failure is acute, chronic, or with acute decompensation of chronic respiratory failure (acute-on-chronic).

- Identify/document the basic disease causing the respiratory failure. Clarify the acute process in relation to a chronic disease (e.g., acute respiratory failure due to pneumonia in a patient with chronic respiratory failure from multiple sclerosis).

- Clarify the presence of hypoxemic or hypercapnic or mixed respiratory failure as appropriate for the patient.

- Document clinical signs, symptoms, and any laboratory findings that support the diagnosis of acute respiratory failure when present.

- Document in the progress notes and discharge summary if the patient had acute respiratory failure upon admission and it resolved.

- Clarify in your documentation if the patient being maintained on a ventilator after a surgical procedure had respiratory failure going into surgery or is being maintained on the ventilator and being managed along with the other disease processes and there is not acute respiratory failure at this time (ventilator management).

Seizures

Conditions in which patients experience seizure activity that do not represent epilepsy exist. Differentiating these from epilepsy is important because a patient's job may depend on such a distinction.

Epilepsy is a condition of recurrent seizures of varying magnitude resulting from the generation of aberrant electrical impulses in the brain. It cannot be cured, but it may respond to medications or, in some cases, surgical intervention.

Types identified include:

- **Petit mal** (may present as stopping in mid-sentence, smacking lips, and/or blinking eyes rapidly, and then resolve)

- **Grand mal** (often tonic-clonic movements of extremities or the whole body)

- **Jacksonian seizures** (marching of tonic activity from one area to another)

- **Partial seizures,** which may be **simple** (without loss of consciousness, lasting 90 seconds or less, with either abnormal sensations or some jerking)

- **Complex** (with loss of consciousness, lasting one to two minutes—differentiated from petit mal by the length of the event)

Most cases of epilepsy (70%–75%) do not have a significant historical event that one can point to and are considered idiopathic. Patients may develop seizure activity during infections of the brain or as a result of scarring in the brain after an infection such as encephalitis, during strokes or as a late effect of strokes because of the healing process of the stroke, with brain neoplasms, or after removal of brain neoplasms because of scarring. When a seizure occurs during the acute event, it is a seizure due to that condition and is not (yet) epilepsy. However, when a patient develops recurring seizures (more than two) linked to these delayed circumstances, this is the hallmark for a diagnosis of epilepsy.

Repeated grand mal seizure activity without significant resolution between seizures is called **status epilepticus;** this can lead to respiratory failure.

An epileptic seizure may be heralded by an aura, and, when of the grand mal variety, may be associated with loss of bowel or bladder function and may be followed by loss of consciousness or amnesia for the event (postictal state).

Mostly in children, fevers can cause seizures called **febrile convulsions.** This is not epilepsy. Simple febrile seizures are generalized convulsions that last less than 15 minutes and do not recur within 24 hours. Complex febrile seizures can be generalized or focal and often last longer than the simple variety but do recur within 24 hours. They are often associated with more serious infections than the usual viral illnesses of children. These seizures may not occur when the temperature is highest and may be the first sign that a viral infection has started.

Seizures can result from lesions in the temporal lobe of the brain, and these may be amenable to surgery if routine antiepileptic medications are not effective (as in the case of temporal lobe epilepsy or mesial temporal sclerosis).

Documentation needs

- Document clearly whether you believe that the patient had a seizure (postictal state) or identify another cause of altered consciousness.

- Document the relationship between other existing diseases (e.g., recent or old stroke, recent or old head trauma, brain tumor, febrile convulsion and whether it was simple or complex, drug overdose, alcoholism, diabetes out of control, viral or other infection, sepsis) and the seizure.

- Identify/document if the patient has hippocampal or mesial temporal sclerosis or other temporal lobe seizure.

- Clearly document whether you determine that a known seizure patient aspirated at the time of the seizure and when the respiratory problem prompted admission.

- Document whether you believe that the patient has epilepsy to differentiate it from other causes of seizure. Identify the type (e.g., simple or complex partial epilepsy, grand mal, petit mal).

- Document whether this event was initially thought to be a seizure and you later determined that it was not a seizure.

Sepsis

Background

Sepsis is a series of chemical and biologic changes in response to an infection that may lead to progressive organ dysfunction and death if not countered by the body's defenses or treated with antibiotics, maintenance of failing organs, and sometimes surgery. Because the risk of mortality is high in patients with severe sepsis, the healthcare industry has published several studies and clinical best practices for treatment protocols and early identification. Physicians, quality leaders, HIM staff, and clinical documentation improvement staff must work closely on the appropriate ways to document sepsis early in the course of treatment. Regulatory audits and reviews of hospital sepsis cases have increased, so documentation must be very specific and detailed. Do not call it sepsis if it's not sepsis and that is your clinical determination.

Bacteremia implies the presence of bacteria in the bloodstream, although not necessarily due to an infection. Bacteremia may exist along with sepsis, or it may be a transient event caused by invasion of the bloodstream from a procedure that led to opening of the bloodstream to a source of infection. This occurs with dental cleanings, which is why patients with heart valve disease receive prophylactic antibiotics for every trip to the dentist, or why patients undergoing transrectal prostate biopsies receive an injection of prophylactic gentamicin or other antibiotic. Currently, infectious disease specialists believe that *bacteremia* is a better term for *septicemia due to bacteria*, *viremia* is a better term for *septicemia due to viruses*, and *fungemia* is a better term for *septicemia due to fungi*. However, reflection of severity of illness is best illustrated with *septicemia, sepsis due to _____*, or *bacteremia with sepsis*.

Septicemia is infection of the bloodstream. Signs and symptoms of septicemia include shaking chills, rigors, temperature spikes, and significantly elevated white blood cell count. It also may coexist with sepsis. With the adoption of ICD-10, there will no longer be a designation for *septicemia*; *bacteremia with sepsis*, *bacterial sepsis*, or *blood stream infection* will be preferred.

A **contaminant** implies that a blood sample was drawn without proper aseptic technique. This permitted growth of an organism on a culture plate, but no infection exists due to that organism.

Colonization implies presence of bacteria in a body orifice or cavity without infection. This often occurs with patients who have indwelling urinary catheters. A positive urine culture in an asymptomatic patient likely represents colonization. Bacteria often colonize tracheostomy stomas and other openings. Patients with bronchiectasis or cystic fibrosis may have colonization with pseudomonas and not have an active infection.

Systemic inflammatory response syndrome (SIRS) is inherent with most infections, and the term should not be used to imply sepsis when sepsis does not exist. Document noninfectious sources of SIRS, such as necrotizing pancreatitis, massive body burns, or large pulmonary emboli.

Criteria of SIRS is not the same as *existence of SIRS*. The criteria are a reflection of changes in vital signs and laboratory results, and imply the syndrome only when they are identified as having been caused by an inflammatory process or by dead tissue.

Documentation needs

- Document in the medical record the source of the infection, if known.

- Document in the medical record the patient's signs and symptoms of sepsis.

- Document the presence of organ failure (e.g., acute renal failure, septic shock, acute respiratory failure, hepatic failure, disseminated intravascular coagulopathy (DIC), critical care myopathy, or metabolic encephalopathy related to sepsis).

- Document whether positive blood cultures are clinically significant or represent contaminants. Remember that absence of positive blood culture does not preclude a sepsis diagnosis.

- Document predisposing factors (e.g., immunocompromise, as in diabetes, steroid therapy, malnutrition, immunoglobulin deficiency, or chemotherapy).

- Document the likelihood of a relationship to implanted devices, such as sepsis or septicemia due to infection of a heart valve (endocarditis), indwelling Foley catheter, or vascular access device.

- Avoid using terms such as *urosepsis* as a substitute for sepsis.

- Specify whether bacteremia is due to a septic condition in the body or is transient due to a procedure or unknown cause.

Stroke or Cerebrovascular Accident

Background

Stroke or cerebrovascular accident (CVA) implies an acute brain event that leads to brain cellular death (infarction) or pressure from a hemorrhage against brain cells that prevents them from functioning properly. Strokes can range in severity from minimal with brief symptoms that resolve in minutes and validated on a subsequent x-ray, to one with sudden loss of consciousness, paralysis, rapid cessation of breathing, and death.

The two major types of stroke are ischemic and hemorrhagic. An **ischemic** stroke may represent an embolism from the heart or from an ulcerated plaque of the carotid artery or a local occlusion of a vessel in the brain. A **hemorrhagic stroke** may be subarachnoid, intracerebral, or intraventricular. Ischemic strokes are identified by the artery involved in the occlusion, if known. Hemorrhagic strokes are identified by the portion of the brain involved with the hemorrhage.

Hemorrhagic strokes are grouped by the lobes of the brain involved; ischemic strokes are grouped by the major intracranial vessel occluded (when known). Both ischemic and hemorrhagic strokes benefit from documentation of which side of the brain was involved (right or left) and whether hemiparesis involved the patient's dominant or nondominant side.

A patient with a **subdural hemorrhage** may have spontaneous or traumatic hemorrhage after a fall and striking the head. For some patients who fall frequently, knowing which occurred first can be difficult.

A transient ischemic attack **(TIA)** is identified as a localizing, lateralizing neurologic deficit that lasts seconds to minutes, such as transient unilateral blindness (amaurosis fugax). It can be caused by a platelet clot that briefly obstructs a vessel in the brain and then breaks apart, after which flow is immediately reestablished, or it can be caused by positional obstruction of an artery to the brain. Vertebrobasilar insufficiency occurs with transient occlusion of blood flow to the cerebellum or base of the brain and may manifest as a fall due to transient vertigo. Sometimes, tight collar syndrome can imitate a carotid TIA and subclavian steal syndrome can present as a vertebrobasilar attack.

If a computed tomography (CT) scan on admission shows an infarct, it is probably an old infarct because, except for massive infarcts, one cannot detect ischemic strokes on CT. CT is performed to determine whether a stroke is hemorrhagic.

Enzymes (such as tissue plasminogen activator) may be administered to a patient with an acute embolic or occlusive stroke if symptoms started within three hours of evaluation and the patient has no other bleeding problems. **Another option is mechanical embolism removal**

in cerebral ischemia (MERCI), which percutaneously removes a clot after embolism if observed within a few hours. Patients admitted with a stroke may have carotid narrowing (carotid stenosis) seen on flow studies. These are not to be construed as causative of the stroke unless a physician makes the link. Often, this is an incidental finding.

Documentation needs

- Document whether you determine that the patient had a hemorrhagic stroke (e.g., intracerebral hemorrhage, subarachnoid hemorrhage; identify the portion of the brain involved) or had an occlusive or embolic cerebral infarction (identify the vessel involved, if known).

- If you diagnose cerebral infarction, document whether it was due to primary intracerebral occlusion (and identify the artery, if possible), carotid disease with embolism from an ulcerated plaque, or cardioembolic stroke.

- Document whether the patient had an evolving stroke that was aborted by enzyme or anticoagulant therapy.

- Document whether the study revealed carotid artery disease as the cause of the patient's current symptoms, and explain whether this hospitalization is because of current cerebral infarction (true stroke) or noninfarction cerebral embolism (TIA).

- Avoid using terms such as *reversible ischemic neurological deficit, cerebrovascular accident,* or only *stroke,* because they may be misconstrued and result in a code assignment that does not represent the true condition.

- Report/document when the patient has clinical signs of increased intracranial pressure, brain shift, herniation (side to side of foramen magnum), spastic or flaccid quadriplegia, and coma. Unresponsiveness does not imply coma when only that condition exists.

- When a patient's family agrees to cease active treatment and let the patient die comfortably, *comfort measures only* is a preferable term to indicate withdrawal of life support or that no further care will be administered, rather than the term *DNR* (do not resuscitate), which implies that all treatment for all conditions will be undertaken to a designated point.

Symptoms

Generally, patients seen in an emergency department or a physician's office exhibit some symptoms. After workup, a diagnosis or several diagnoses may be identified as the cause of the symptoms. For capturing clinical data and for billing purposes, symptoms are used for billing to justify studies done. In a hospital, diagnoses after workup are preferable to capture significant patient information, and the link of the diagnoses to those presenting symptoms is paramount to ensure the proper sequencing of codes.

When a patient is admitted for signs and symptoms and a diagnosis is never established, that which you believe to be the cause takes precedence. Sometimes there is no way to determine the cause of the signs and symptoms, so the sign or symptom becomes the principal diagnosis.

When signs and symptoms of an adverse effect of a prescription drug occur, the sign or symptom is the principal diagnosis.

Documentation needs

- Document distinctly the relationship between signs and symptoms on admission and the diagnoses determined after workup

- If a symptom may be due to either of two (or more) diagnoses, clearly document this information

- If a patient's symptoms could be due to several diseases, none of which you are sure the patient has, clearly document this information

- Document the diagnosis that you believe exists whenever you order studies or treatments while a patient is in the hospital

Note: For cardiac arrest or cardiorespiratory arrest, document the most likely cause of the event (e.g., acute MI, Takotsubo syndrome, ventricular tachycardia/fibrillation, stroke, sepsis with shock). If you cannot determine the cause, that is fine.

Syncope

Syncope or fainting is usually due to decreased blood flow to the brain, whether cardiogenic or neurogenic in origin. Certain historical events point to a likely cause of syncope or near syncope.

This must be differentiated from other clinical conditions, such as a fall from tripping or a history of repeated falls due to normal pressure hydrocephalus, muscular weakness due to stroke or as a late effect of a previous stroke, transient ischemic attacks (TIA) (especially posterior circulation of the brain), malnutrition with weakness, brain tumors, subarachnoid bleeds, or other strokes.

Common causes of **cardiogenic syncope** include bradycardia, tachycardia with reduced diastolic filling of the heart, symptomatic aortic stenosis (including hypertrophic obstructive cardiomyopathy), venous pooling as from tight belt syndrome, hypovolemia as can occur with severe dehydration, or massive hemorrhagic events (e.g., gastrointestinal bleed, menorrhagia, ruptured aneurysm).

Neurogenic syncope includes vasovagal responses (such as after seeing something horrifying), rapid emptying of the bowels or bladder (called postmicturition syncope), adverse effect of beta-blockers, primary autonomic nerve dysfunction, diabetic neuropathy.

The clinician first must rule out acute MI, stroke, and sepsis.

Orthostatic vital signs, or increase in heart rate and drop in blood pressure when changing from supine to sitting or sitting to standing, is not the same as the disease **orthostatic hypotension.** Orthostatic drop in blood pressure with testing can be a clinical sign of a vast number of diseases, including most of those previously mentioned. True orthostatic hypotension usually represents adrenal insufficiency or primary autonomic neuropathy. Look for a disease from the previous paragraphs to explain the syncope.

Documentation needs

- If a patient experiences an identifiable event, such as postmicturition syncope, cough-related syncope, frightening event, or sudden positional change, identify it in the medical record as the cause of the syncope

- If causative dehydration, arrhythmia, or drug–drug interaction occurred, identify and document the cause

- If a patient tripped and fell, document it in the medical record instead of calling it syncope when it wasn't

- If a patient had an AMI, stroke, or sepsis, identify and document the condition as the cause of the syncopal episode

- If a patient had acute cerebrovascular insufficiency signs of chronic cerebrovascular ischemia with an acute insufficiency event, identify and document it as the cause of the episode

Trauma

Background

Many visits to the emergency department are due to traumatic events. The appropriate designation of the damage to the body often depends on proper documentation that will lead to the code that tells the same story. Furthermore, trauma teams are developed in hospitals to address multiple significant traumas. This particular group of patients is often tracked statistically within a group of cases that involve significant trauma to at least three body systems. Multiple broken bones constitute one body system, unless one of them is the skull and another includes at least six ribs.

Closed head injury can result in a laceration of the scalp or the brain, skull or facial bone fracture, or contusion or hemorrhage to the brain. It is inadequate to merely call it closed head injury unless no other damage was identified. Specifying cerebral concussion, cerebral contusion, or cerebral hemorrhage has major implications for severity of a trauma case.

Specifying presence of unconsciousness or coma is important, as is identifying how long the patient was unconscious, if known, and whether the patient is expected to awaken. Assigning a Glasgow coma score to a patient indicates severity of the brain damage. It can be computed at the site of the injury by the emergency medical services team, upon arrival in the emergency department, and upon admission to the hospital. These are codable either by individual elements of the coma scores or by cumulative numbers.

Documentation needs

- Document the presence or history of cerebral concussion or cause of transient loss of consciousness, even if resolved by the time you see the patient.

- Document known evaluations of Glasgow coma scores and locations and times that they were evaluated.

- Document whether the patient had hypovolemia or hypovolemic shock in the presence of bleed or multiple bone fractures on admission.

- Document the number of fractured ribs on each side (total number of ribs fractured).

- Document the fracture or dislocation of each bone and whether it was treated by stabilization or surgery or not treated at all. Do not identify fractures by joint involved unless the fracture also goes through the joint.

- Document when a patient has pulmonary contusion with or without respiratory failure.

- Identify the cause (e.g., bilateral tension hemopneumothorax, fat embolism, pulmonary contusion, shock, lung aspiration pneumonitis, upper cervical vertebral fracture with spinal cord injury, alcohol or drug abuse) if the patient has acute respiratory failure.

- Include all diagnoses established from admission of the trauma case through discharge.

Refer to Figure 4 for information about the Glasgow Coma Scale.

Figure 4: Glasgow Coma System of Scoring

Category		Best Response
Eye opening		
Spontaneous		4
To speech		3
To pain		2
None		1
Verbal	(Modified for Infants)	
Oriented	Babbles	5
Confused	Irritable	4
Inappropriate words	Cries to pain	3
Moans	Moans	2
None	None	1
Motor		
Follows commands		6
Localizes to pain		5
Withdraws to pain		4
Abnormal flexion		3
Abnormal extension		2
None		1
Glasgow Coma Scale		
Best possible score		15
Worst possible score		3
If tracheally intubated then verbal designated with "T"		
Best possible score while intubated		10T
Worst possible score while intubated		2T

Summary

The emphasis on clinical documentation improvement and precision is ongoing and will continue. Many reasons, rationales, and benefits are associated with ensuring complete, specific, and detailed documentation in a patient's medical record. Physicians and the healthcare community can work together to bring greater awareness and attention to capturing patient severity of illness and risk of mortality.

The community and holistic approach to healthcare delivery make the ability of data to represent a patient's health status paramount. With incomplete documentation, other healthcare workers will be unable to identify what is missing from a patient's list of current chronic and/or acute diagnoses, and the patient will suffer.

Some next steps that can be undertaken include:

- Improvements or enhancements to the electronic health record. Templates and smart phrases may also be helpful with appropriate review and use.

- Physician community awareness of clinical documentation needs for proper ICD and CPT® code assignment.

- Shared scorecard and profile data.

- Engagement in the coding process and work of the coding staff.

- Collaboration with clinical documentation improvement (CDI) staff.

- Greater communication and dialogue between compliance, quality, risk, health information management, CDI, and medical staff.

With greater attention to the topics discussed in this book and with enhanced communication and collaboration, providers can benefit from improved patient care, outcomes, and appropriate reimbursement. Now is the time to work together and make a difference.

NOTES

NOTES

NOTES

NOTES